Contemporary Cardiovascular Disease Risk Factors in Special Populations™

Ezra A. Amsterdam, MD
Professor of Internal Medicine and Associate Director,
Division of Cardiovascular Medicine,
University of California, Davis, School of Medicine, Sacramento, CA

JoAnne M. Foody, MD, FACC, FAHA
Associate Professor, Harvard Medical School,
Brigham and Women's/Faulkner Hospitals, Boston, MA

C. Tissa Kappagoda, MD, PhD
Professor, Department of Internal Medicine,
Director, Coronary Heart Disease Reversal Program, and
Director, Cardiac Rehabilitation Program,
University of California, Davis, School of Medicine, Sacramento, CA

Philip R. Liebson, MD
Professor of Medicine and Preventive Medicine, Associate Director,
Section of Cardiology, McMullan-Eybel Chair of Excellence in Cardiology
Rush University Medical Center, Chicago, IL

First Edition

Published by Handbooks in Health Care Co.,
Newtown, Pennsylvania, USA

This book is not intended to replace or to be used as a substitute for the complete prescribing information prepared by each manufacturer for each drug. Because of possible variations in drug indications, in dosage information, in newly described toxicities, in drug/drug interactions, and in other items of importance, reference to such complete prescribing information is definitely recommended before any of the drugs discussed are used or prescribed.

International Standard Book Number: 978-1-935103-21-9

Library of Congress Catalog Card Number: 2009942978

Authors and Contributors

This book has been prepared and is presented as a service to the medical community. The information provided reflects the knowledge, experience, and personal opinions of lead authors, Philip R. Liebson, MD, Professor of Medicine and Preventive Medicine, The McMullan Eybel Chair of Excellence in Cardiology, Rush University Medical Center, Chicago, Illinois; C. Tissa Kappagoda, MD, PhD, Professor, Director of Coronary Heart Disease Reversal Program, Director of Cardiac Rehabilitation Program, University of California, Davis, School of Medicine, Sacramento, California; JoAnne M. Foody, MD, Associate Professor, Harvard Medical School, Brigham and Women's/ Faulkner Hospitals, Boston, Massachusetts; and Ezra A. Amsterdam, MD, Professor of Internal Medicine and Associate Director, Division of Cardiovascular Medicine, University of California, Davis, School of Medicine, Sacramento, California. The information provided also reflects the knowledge, experience, and personal opinions of the contributing authors, L. Veronica Lee, MD, Assistant Professor of Medicine, Division of Cardiovascular Medicine, Yale University, New Haven, Connecticut, and Laura L. Hayman, PhD, RN, Associate Dean for Research, Professor of Nursing, College of Nursing and Health Sciences, University of Massachusetts, and Director of Research, GoKids, Boston.

Table of Contents

Chapter 1

Scope of the Problem

By Philip R. Liebson, MD

Health-care providers today need to emphasize the disparities in the prevention, presence, and treatment of cardiovascular disease (CVD) among people of different races, ethnic groups, and gender, and appreciate the importance of socioeconomic, cultural, and geographic considerations. Focusing on these disparities in special populations may lead to better health protection catered to these differences. Evidence is increasing that the approaches to diagnosis and treatment of CVD between men and women are different, and it is only recently that the primacy of CVD in women, as well as men, has been widely recognized. In regard to race or ethnicity, the differences in prevalence and treatment of risk and CVD in whites, blacks, Hispanics, Native Americans, and Asians deserve clarification. We hope that this concise handbook will provide a perspective on these differences to assist health-care professionals in implementing CVD prevention and treatment in these special populations.

In this book, for simplicity, we use the terms black, white, Hispanic, and Asian most often, although Caucasian, African American, Mexican American, Native American, South Asian, and East Asian are regularly used in many relevant studies. Perhaps in another century any of these terms will be considered quaint when more knowledge about genetics is uncovered, but for now there are clear-cut differences in characteristics of comorbidities, risk factors, mortality, and disease management features among these groups. Understanding those differences is the rationale for this book. We use the term *gender* because it is used most often in study nomenclature, even though we are aware that this is a grammatical construct and that the term *sex* is more appropriate to differentiate males and females.

This introduction provides an overview of some of the considerations involved in these differences, establishing a basis for separate chapters on women and on topics focusing on racial/ethnic implications, continuous risk factors, and CVD patterns.

A recent report of the American Heart Association (AHA) Statistics Committee and Stroke Statistics Committee provides important ethnic and gender differences in heart disease and stroke in the United States[1] (Appendix A). Heart disease prevalence varies considerably among ethnic groups, from 6.7% in those of Asian ethnicity to 12%-13% in whites and American Indians.[1] For example, the overall death rate from CVD varies from 238/100,000 in white women to 454/100,000 in black men. Comparing ethnicity and gender differences in one ethnic group, in persons 45 to 64 years of age, the age-adjusted incidence of coronary events varies from 4.0/1,000 person-years in white women to 12.5/1,000 in white men.[1]

An example of outcomes of a significant risk factor between ethnic groups for CVD is provided by the San Luis Valley Diabetes Study (1984-1998), which compared non-Hispanic whites and Hispanics in a community. The CVD and coronary heart disease (CHD) death rate ratios were significantly lower in Hispanic men with diabetes in comparison with non-Hispanic white male diabetics without significant ethnic differences in rate ratios among diabetic women and nondiabetic men and women.[2] Mortality rate ratios of Hispanic diabetic males compared with non-Hispanic diabetic males was 0.42 for CVD mortality and 0.34 for coronary artery disease (CAD) mortality.[2]

Marked differences are seen in lifestyle risk factors. For example, in 2005, 6.1% of women of Asian ethnicity more than 17 years of age were cigarette smokers compared to 37.5% of American-Indian men.[1] Early lifestyle differences are also marked. In 2005, the prevalence of high school students meeting recommended levels of physical activity during the previous week varied from 21% in black girls to 47% in white boys. In the same group, the percentage of overweight adolescents varied from 8.2% in white girls to 16.1% in black girls.[1] These and other statistics indicate the considerable variations in risk factors in special populations and have important implications for the occurrence of CVD in these groups.

Some disparities are particularly outstanding. For example, in the current epidemic of obesity, compilations of national surveys in the US evaluating gender, ethnicity, and socioeconomic and geographic differences indicate that obesity—a risk factor for diabetes, lipid abnormalities, and hypertension—all of which are risk factors for CVD—are most common in Mexican-American men with a high school education (29%) and in black women without a high school education (47%).[3] This finding and other differences may explain the disparities among ethnic groups in death rates from CVD and the years of potential life lost. For example, from the Behavioral Risk Factor Surveillance System 1990, 1996, and 2003 analyses, blacks (per 100,000 persons) had 2,249 years of potential life lost to diseases of the heart, 1,261 years lost to ischemic heart disease, and 491 years lost to stroke, compared with 1,115 years, 773 years, and 176 years for whites, respectively. Asians and Pacific Islanders were lowest of ethnic groups, with 547 years, 369 years, and 198 years lost, respectively.[3] Clinicians must also consider the importance of socioeconomic differences that can lead to CVD, such as poverty status, education, and income levels.[3]

In terms of medical care, hospitalization is greater for men for heart disease and acute myocardial infarction (MI) and greater for women for congestive heart failure (CHF) and stroke. In older age groups (Medicare enrollees), whites have fewer hospitalizations for CHF than do blacks, Hispanics, and Native Americans.[3] In terms of geography, hospitalization for stroke and CHF is highest in the southeast.

As for outcomes, CVD mortality is higher among blacks than for other racial and ethnic groups. In 2001, it was 30% higher in blacks compared to non-Hispanic whites.[4] Life expectancy is higher in women than in men, and in whites compared to blacks, each by 5 years. These are only a few of the differences that require consideration in terms of genetic and environmental influences on disease and risk factors, selection for hospitalization and intervention, and intensity of recurrent medical evaluations.

The Third National Health and Nutrition Examination Survey (NHANES III) from 1988-1994 evaluated elderly white, Mexican-American, and black men and women in relation to CVD risk factors, and found a higher prevalence of diabetes in Mexican-American and black women than in white women, after adjustment for age and socioeconomic status[5] (Tables 1-1 to 1-3). Physical inactivity and hypertension were more likely in blacks than in whites in both women and men (Table 1-2). Ethnicity was associated significantly with CVD risk factors in logistic regression models. Differences in health behaviors in attempts to reduce risk vary considerably (Table 1-3). Non-high-density lipoprotein cholesterol (non-HDL-C), an important CVD risk factor, was higher in black than white women.

These examples of differences in the burden of risk factors, outcomes, and disease management underline the importance of increased CVD risk in ethnic minority populations and the special attention needed for gender differences. Moreover, cultural and language differences must be considered in efforts to improve medical care and disease prevention. The examples indicate that important ethnic and gender comparisons should include investigation of CVD risk factors, pathophysiologic and metabolic differ-

Table 1-1: Sample Sizes, Sociodemographic, and Health-Care Considerations by Gender and Ethnicity, Women and Men, Ages 65-84, NHANES III, 1988-1994

	Women				Men			
	Black	Mexican-American	White		Black	Mexican-American	White	
US population (millions)[a]	1.3	0.3	13.2		0.9	0.3	10.3	
Analytic sample[b]	352	307	1124		348	321	1068	
Sociodemographic characteristics[c]								
Age, mean, yr	72.4	70.5	73.1		71.6	71.4	72.0	
% currently married	27.2	48.1	45.7		62.8	82.7	79.9	
% living in urban area	49.2	50.3	39.7		50.8	47.3	41.9	
% below poverty level	37.8	37.6	10.1		27.3	29.8	5.0	
Education, mean, yr	9.1	5.3	11.4		8.6	5.7	11.6	

10

% born abroad	2.7	41.9	4.9	3.5	36.6	4.1
% speaking Spanish at home	1.0	69.8	2.3	1.5	73.0	2.6
Health-care characteristics[c]						
% reporting medical insurance	98.2	96.9	99.9	98.9	96.0	99.6
% with particular clinic, health center, or doctor's office to go to if sick or need advice	94.0	90.1	93.5	88.4	84.6	90.1
% with one particular doctor or health professional who is usually seen	86.4	78.0	90.2	74.1	73.6	83.2
Times seen a doctor or assistant in last 12 mo, mean	6.9	5.2	4.8	4.2	5.1	4.4

[a]Projected estimates based on weighted percentages from NHANES III defined sample.
[b]Number who participated in both the home questionnaire and medical examination, unweighed.
[c]Means and averages were calculated with normalized sample weights.
Used with permission from the American Geriatrics Society © 2001. From Sundquist[5]

11

Table 1-2: Pravalences of Cardiovascular Risk Factors by Gender and Ethnicity, Ages 65-84, NHANES III[a], 1988-1994[b]

	Type 2 Diabetes (%)	Physical Inactivity (%)	Abdominal Obesity (%)
Women			
Black	28.1	48.1	76.2
Mexican-American	32.6	39.5	65.2
Whites	17.0	30.8	66.0
Men			
Black	19.1	27.7	34.1
Mexican-American	19.7	26.3	36.8
Whites	15.5	17.1	46.6

[a]NHANES III=Third National Health and Nutrition Examination Survey.
[b]Percentages were calculated with normalized sample weights adjusted for age and education.
[c]Non-HDL-C=non-high-density lipoprotein cholesterol.

ences in the presence and distribution of CVD, and efforts to implement risk reduction and CVD modification.

Disease and Risk Patterns

A characteristic example of ethnic differences is the higher CHD mortality in blacks compared to non-Hispanic whites.[6-8] A partial explanation may be the higher

Hypertension (%)	Current Smoking (%)	High Non-HDL Cholesterol[c] (%)
74.1	10.4	59.0
71.7	11.7	69.0
62.0	10.7	69.8
67.1	20.2	49.2
51.2	11.9	53.9
52.6	15.4	56.1

From Sundquist J,[5] with permission.

prevalence, in blacks, of risk factors such as hypertension and diabetes, target-organ damage such as left ventricular hypertrophy (LVH), and chronic renal failure,[9,10] as well as differences in intervention once CHD develops.[10,11]

The differences in classical risk factors in various ethnic groups have been increasingly evaluated, especially in regard to Hispanics and blacks versus non-Hispanic

Table 1-3: Health Behavior and Compliance With Doctors' Recommendations Among Those With Type 2 Diabetes, Abdominal Obesity, Hypertension, High Blood Cholesterol, and Those who Smoke, by Gender and Ethnicity, Ages 65-84, NHANES III,[a] 1988-1994[b]

	Type II Diabetes	
	Checked urine or blood for sugar at least once/mo (%)	Had eyes dilated within past 2 yr (%)
Women		
Black	36.6	59.3
Mexican-American	22.1	42.0
English-speaking	37.4	51.7
Spanish-speaking	16.9	38.7
White	53.7	58.3
Men[c]		
Black	55.8	50.8
Mexican-American	47.1	63.6
White	52.7	67.8

[a]NHANES III=Third National Health and Nutrition Examination Survey.
[b]Percentages calculated with normalized sample weights.
BP=blood pressure, C=cholesterol
From Sundquist J,[5] with permission.

Abdominal Obesity		Current Smoking
Tried to lose weight in past 12 mo (%)	Changed diet for medical reasons past 12 mo (%)	Tried to quit smoking in past 12 mo (%)
46.2	31.3	22.8
37.1	27.6	35.7
54.3	40.9	66.4
31.1	23.0	20.0
49.0	27.0	26.4
43.4	25.3	23.5
37.9	16.2	37.4
41.7	19.5	24.2

ᶜThere were too few English-speaking Mexican-American men to examine health behaviors by language spoken.

Note: Significant differences between ethnic groups $P <0.001$ and $P <0.05$

(continued on next page)

Table 1-3: Health Behavior and Compliance With Doctors' Recommendations Among Those With Type 2 Diabetes, Abdominal Obesity, Hypertension, High Blood Cholesterol, and Those who Smoke, by Gender and Ethnicity, Ages 65-84, NHANES III,[a] 1988-1994[b] *(continued)*

	Hypertension		
	Compliance with physician's recommendation to:		
	Take prescribed medicine for high BP (%)	Control or lose weight for high BP (%)	Use less salt or sodium for high BP (%)
Women			
Black	89.4	86.3	93.7
Mexican-American	76.0	82.0	91.1
English-speaking	81.3	79.0	92.7
Spanish-speaking	74.3	83.3	90.6
White	86.3	78.1	93.4
Men[c]			
Black	83.2	92.1	96.3
Mexican-American	87.0	89.1	97.1
White	82.4	76.5	92.4

[a]NHANES III=Third National Health and Nutrition Examination Survey.

[b]Percentages calculated with normalized sample weights.

BP=blood pressure, C=cholesterol

High Blood Cholesterol

Compliance with physician's recommendation to:

Eat fewer high-fat foods for high BP (%)	Lose weight to lower C (%)	Exercise to lower C (%)	Take prescribed medicine to lower C (%)
94.9	89.6	84.8	90.4
95.9	96.4	75.2	45.9
96.0	100.0	83.8	46.5
95.8	94.9	69.0	45.5
95.8	87.2	79.2	73.2
93.5	100.0	97.8	91.7
84.0	98.2	85.4	91.7
90.0	83.3	76.2	77.7

ᶜThere were too few English-speaking Mexican-American men to examine health behaviors by language spoken.

Note: Significant differences between ethnic groups $P < 0.001$ and $P < 0.05$

whites. The NHANES evaluations provided important information on such differences. For example, based on NHANES IV (1998-2004), using multiple logistic regression, the probability of being hypertensive was assessed for participants 15 to 65 years of age.[12] Black to white odds for development of hypertension increased from 1.71 to 3.12 between ages 15 to 65, with odds for black women increasing faster (2.11-4.04). Adjustment for poverty income did not affect these results, but adjustment for body mass index (BMI) reduced black women's hypertension risk but not black men's.

Data from NHANES IV in various age groups indicated modest differences in total cholesterol in whites, blacks, and Mexican Americans in the 12- to 19-year age group, the lowest in white adolescent males (157.1 mg/dL), and the highest in white adolescent females (167.5 mg/dL).[1] Similarly, low-density lipoprotein cholesterol (LDL-C) levels in that age group varied between 87.9 mg/dL in black males up to 92.0 mg/dL in Mexican-American females. NHANES data for HDL-C in this young population indicated more of a scatter, the lowest average value being 47.0 mg/dL in white males and the highest 57.6 mg/dL in black females. NHANES data in persons in these three ethnic categories over the age of 20 demonstrated few differences in percentage of LDL-C values above 130 mg/dL (from 29.8% in black women to 33.8 % in white women), but the percentage of persons with HDL-C levels <40 mg/dL varied considerably. The highest percentage of low of HDL-C was found in Mexican-American males (27.7%) and the lowest in black females (6.9%). Black males had the lowest percentage of low HDL-C levels (15.5% vs 26%-27% in males of the other two ethnicities).

Trends in total cholesterol from the National Center for Health Statistics indicate a decrease in total cholesterol from 1976-1980 to 2003-2004 in adolescent boys and girls of both black and white ethnicity, from a mean of 166 to 160 mg/dL in whites and from 171 to 161 mg/dL in blacks.[1]

In white, black, and Mexican-American adults there has been a similar decrease from 1988-1994 to 2003-2004, varying from -4 mg/dL in whites and Mexican Americans to -7 mg/dL in blacks.

Several other studies have documented differences in lipoprotein levels in younger ethnic groups. The Coronary Artery Risk Development in Young Adults (CARDIA) study in a biracial population (black and white) 23 to 35 years of age found that the prevalence of LDL-C levels >160 mg/dL varied between 4% in white women to 10% in black men.[13] Similarly, the prevalence of HDL-C <35 mg/dL varied from 3% in women, 7% in black men, and 13% in white men.

In the Bogalusa Heart Study, lipid data in young adults 20 to 37 years of age demonstrated that whites had significantly higher levels of very-low-density lipoprotein (VLDL), $VLDL_3$, and LDL, and lower levels of HDL_2 and HDL_3 than did blacks.[14] The significance of genetic influences appeared to vary biracially. Positive parental history of CAD was associated significantly with LDL in white males and HDL_2 and LDL_3 (small, dense) lipoproteins in white females, but there was no relationship in blacks. Earlier studies had demonstrated mean HDL-C levels almost 10 mg/dL higher in black than white adult males aged 20 to 44.[15] Associated were lower triglyceride levels, which reduced but did not eliminate the significance of the increased HDL-C. The adjusted mean differences were lower in black children (+2.9 mg/dL) and increased in adults (+7.9 mg/dL).

There is ample evidence that obesity and diabetes are epidemic in the US, with a considerable increase in both over the last two decades. These disorders are important elements of the metabolic syndrome, a strong risk factor for cardiovascular events. The syndrome involves characteristics of blood pressure, lipid values, waist circumference, and blood glucose levels. Data from 1988-1994 NHANES III among whites, blacks, and Mexican Americans indicated variation in prevalence from 13.9% in black men to 27.2% in Mexican-American women.[1] The more stringent guidelines for blood glucose and the increase in weight in the general US population since that survey suggest that the prevalence of metabolic syndrome may have increased significantly in recent years. The more recent data from NHANES IV and the National Health Interview Survey covering 2001 through 2005 indicate a very high percentage in these three ethnic groups of overweight (from 58% in white women to 80% in black women).[1] In terms of plasma glucose, a similar survey of whites, blacks, and Mexican Americans from 1999 to 2004 evaluating the prevalence of diabetes and prediabetes indicated a variation from 29% in white women to almost 50% in Mexican-American men. A recent study of the impact of ethnicity and the metabolic syndrome on the presence of CHD conducted at two New York State medical centers evaluated blacks and whites undergoing coronary angiography.[16] The overall prevalence of the metabolic syndrome was high in both groups (65.5% in whites and 29.1% in blacks), far higher than in the general population. Those with the metabolic syndrome had a far higher percentage of significant CAD in both ethnic groups. For example, 24% to 31% of white men and women without the metabolic syndrome had evidence for CAD compared with 69% to 76% in those with the metabolic syndrome. Similar differences were found with black women, but paradoxically, black men without the metabolic syndrome had a higher prevalence of CAD than those with the metabolic syndrome (55% vs 45%). These results indicate the association of the metabolic syndrome with significant coronary atherosclerosis in both ethnic groups but that differences in the impact of the metabolic syndrome may vary among ethnic groups.

One of the components of metabolic syndrome, waist circumference, is an important measure of abdominal adiposity. Data from 10,969 participants of NHANES III indicated that waist circumference was a better indicator of CVD risk than BMI in blacks, whites, and Mexican Americans.[17] The odds ratio for having one or more CVD risk factor diverged among ethnic groups for both men and women with respect to BMI and waist circumference. Initiation of divergence was seen in waist circumference above 100 cm (39 in) in men and 86 cm (34 in) in women. The greatest increase in risk of CVD risk factors above these values was found with Hispanic men compared with other men, and white women compared with other women. For example, at a waist circumference of 136 cm (53.5 in), the odds ratio for CVD risk factors had more than an 18-fold increase compared with the lowest waist circumference values, compared with a 14-fold increase in black men and a 12-fold increase in white men. On the other hand, at a waist circumference of 126 cm (49.6 in), the highest odds ratio increase from the lowest waist circumference was 19-fold in white women, but only 10-fold in Hispanic women, and less than 6-fold in black women. These differences should not detract from the importance of waist circumference increase as a CVD risk factor in all groups.

Socioeconomic Status

Education and economic considerations are related to risk differences among various ethnic groups. For example, the third NHANES Survey (1988-1994) of the US population used educational level as a proxy for socioeconomic status (SES).[18] The relationship between ethnicity and absence of CVD risk factors varied within three levels of education. Blacks were twice as likely as other groups to have four or five risk factors for CVD. Among all groups, the prevalence of no risk factors increased with educational status (6%-14% among those with <12 years education to 22% to 29% among those with >12 years education [college level]). However, even in these two groups, ethnic differences were present. In those with <12 years of education, Mexican Americans were 60% more likely and blacks 30% less likely to have no risk factors than did whites. In those with higher education, Mexican Americans and blacks were 50% to 60% less likely to have no risk factors compared with whites.

The same NHANES survey found that most CVD risk factors were higher among ethnic minority women than white women.[19] In women from lower SES, whatever the ethnic group, significantly higher prevalence of smoking and physical inactivity and higher levels of BMI and non-HDL-C were found compared to those with higher SES (Figure 1-1).

The impact of SES in a high-risk black population for diabetes may be less than expected and perhaps genetic influences may be more important. An intriguing study from Ohio State Medical Center evaluated 200 first-degree relatives of black patients with type 2 diabetes. In assessing CVD risk factors, no differences were found in lipid values, insulin levels, glucose levels, or C-peptide levels through quartiles of income (<$20,000 to >$50,000), nor were there differences in lipid levels.[20] It is possible that the income grouping was not broad enough to evaluate effects of much higher income.

On the other hand, an assessment of possible racial disparities in an analysis of 34,331 black and 9,491 white adults with type 2 diabetes recruited from a southern community cohort demonstrated that with similar SES and similar risk factor profiles, no significant differences in diabetes prevalence were found.[21] The study also did not find a more detrimental effect among blacks for obesity compared with whites.

Inflammatory processes may be increased in patients with lower SES because of increased smoking, obesity, alcohol use, and decreased physical activity. The mediating effects of inflammation on atherosclerosis are well studied. For example, the recent Multi-ethnic Study of Atherosclerosis (MESA), which included SES and evaluated the presence of inflammation in a multiethnic population, provided insights into its role in ethnic variation of atherogenesis.[22] Low levels of education and income were associated with higher levels of interleukin-6 and C-reactive protein (CRP, a suspected culprit in atherogenesis) among both whites and

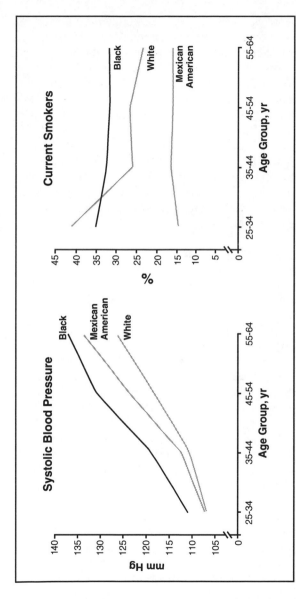

Figure 1-1: From NHANES III, 1988-1994. Significant interactions between ethnicity and age for blood pressure and smoking in women 25 to 64 years of age. From Winkleby[19] with permission from the American Medical Association © 1998.

blacks. However, adiposity was the single most important factor linked to socioeconomic associations, with a smaller effect for psychosocial factors and behavioral patterns in all racial groups, which included Hispanics and Chinese.

A recent study showed that blacks, Hispanics, and women are more likely to have high levels of CRP.[23] The fourth NHANES survey (1999-2004) examined the association of SES and CRP in 7,634 US adults. No significant differences were noted by SES for moderate (1.1-3.0 mg/L) or high (3.0-10.0 mg/L) levels of CRP, but very high levels (>10.0 mg/L) were found more often in those with income at or below poverty level (15.7%) than in those above poverty level (9.1%), with the previously noted gender and ethnic differences.

Community Management

The excessive risk of black subjects with a family history of premature CHD, discussed at the beginning of this chapter, was a stimulus for a community-based (Baltimore), multiple risk factor prevention to reduce CHD risk in high-risk black families study.[24] Black siblings, 30 to 59 years of age of probands with premature CHD, were randomized for modification of classic risk factors into two groups: community-based care or enhanced primary care. The former involved care at a nonclinical site using a nurse practitioner and community health worker. The enhanced primary care involved management in a physician's office. The community-based approach led to a two-fold increase in achievement of blood pressure and lipid goals compared with enhanced primary care, with a significant reduction in global CHD risk, versus no reduction in the enhanced primary care group. This underscores the efficacy of community-based approaches, such as church-based blood pressure evaluations, in blacks. Access to care is important in all ethnic groups, of course, and considerations of travel, appointment times, and the need to care for children during visits are other factors that can pose as barriers to adequate access. The community-based approach used a safe environment, easily accessible by subway and bus for many, and within walking distance of home for many others. An exercise room with a choice of music and a children's play area were provided. Appointments were not necessary and evening and Saturday appointments were available in addition to the daily weekday schedule.

One of the changes in the physician's office environment that this author has seen over the last 40 years is the reduction of the rigid environment in the office. Young children and other members of the family are now routinely brought in to the examining room with the patient, and although the physical examination is usually conducted in the absence of these members, their presence during the patient interview and discussion of therapy frequently assists in implementing management and educating the family on matters of risk. This kind of flexible office environment and the enhancement of community facilities in risk factor modification promise to lead to substantial decreases in risk over the next few decades.

Summary

In 2003, an AHA conference on minority health focused on some of the issues relevant to our discussion.[4] Ethnic diversity is increasing in the US to the extent that non-Hispanic whites may comprise less than a majority of the US population by mid-century. Hispanics now represent 15% of the population and blacks approximately 12%. With the expected increase in the minority proportion of the population, the issues discussed in this chapter take on increasing importance. The evidence that blacks and Hispanics are less likely to undergo interventional cardiac procedures, whether influenced by ethnic or socioeconomic factors, indicates disparities in the health-care delivery system that need rectification.

In terms of genetics, although at least 15 million genetic polymorphisms exist within the human genome,[4] certain ones may be particularly relevant to blacks. For example, aside from the β-globulin (sickle) gene, others include factor V Leiden mutation, leading to increased thrombosis and genes influencing renal sodium channels, leading to increased salt sensitivity and hypertension. Other genes that may have an impact on blacks, leading to CVD risk, include an increase in a mineralocorticoid receptor activator gene and alleles for genes increasing risk for LVH. Differences in levels of circulating nitric oxide and higher levels of superoxide in healthy black women compared to white women also may affect the risk for inflammation and atherogenesis.

Nonetheless, the impact of lifestyle factors cannot be underestimated, as demonstrated by the markedly high percentage of overweight or obese black women >40 years of age (perhaps as much as 80%) and the differences in heart disease prevalence in persons of Japanese ancestry living in Japan, Hawaii, and San Francisco reported in the Honolulu Heart Program.

Overcoming communication barriers is critically important in the implementation of successful management of preventive measures. Community outreach centers have demonstrated effective approaches to modification of lifestyle in certain ethnic groups in comparison to office practice. Appropriate transcultural awareness by health professionals goes a long way to effective management of CVD in special populations and fosters competence in dealing with disease and its prevention.

References

1.   Rosamond W, Flegal K, Furie K, et al, for the American Heart Association Statistics Committee and Stroke Statistics Subcommittee: Heart Disease and Stroke Statistics 2008 update: A report from the American Heart Association Statistics Committee and Stroke Statistics Subcommittee. *Circulation* 2008;117;e25-e146.

2.   Swenson CJ, Trepka MJ, Rewers MJ, et al: Cardiovascular disease mortality in Hispanics and non-Hispanic whites. *Am J Epidemiol* 2002;156:919-928.

3. Mensah GA, Mokdad AH, Ford ES, et al: State of disparities of cardiovascular health in the United States. *Circulation* 2005;111:1233-1241.

4. Yancey CW, Benjamin EJ, Fabunmi RP, et al: Discovering the full spectrum of cardiovascular disease: Minority Health Summit 2005: executive summary. *Circulation* 2005;111:1339-1349.

5. Sundquist J, Winkleby MA, Pudaric S: Cardiovascular disease risk factors among older black, Mexican-American, and white women and men: an analysis of NHANES III, 1988-1994. Third National Health and Nutrition Examination Survey. *J Am Geriatr Soc* 2001;49:109-116.

6. Manolio TA, Burke GL, Psaty M, et al: Black-white differences in subclinical cardiovascular disease among older adults; the cardiovascular health study: CHS collaborative research group. *J Clin Epidemiol* 1995;48:1141-1152.

7. Liao Y, Cooper RS: Continued adverse trends in coronary heart disease mortality among blacks, 1980-91. *Public Health Rep* 1995;110:572-579.

8. Williams JE, Massing M, Rosamond, et al: Racial disparities in CHD mortality from 1968-1992 in the state economic areas surrounding the ARIC study communities: Atherosclerosis Risk in Communities. *Ann Epidemiol* 1999;9:472-480.

9. Harris MI, Flegal KM, Cowie CC, et al: Prevalence of diabetes, impaired fasting glucose, and impaired glucose tolerance in U.S adults. *Diabetes Care* 1998;21:518-524.

10. Davis SK, Liu Y, Gibbons GH: Disparities in trends of hospitalization for potentially preventable chronic conditions among African Americans during the 1990s: implications and benchmarks. *Am J Public Health* 2003;93:447-455.

11. Ghali JK, Cooper RS, Kowatly I, et al: Delay between onset of chest pain and arrival to the coronary care unit among minority and disadvantaged patients. *J Natl Med Assoc* 1993;85:180-184.

12. Geronimus AST, Bound J, Keene D, et al: Black-white differences in age trajectories of hypertension prevalence among adult men and women, 1999-2002. *Ethnic Dis* 2007;17:40-48.

13. Gidding SS, Liu K, Bild DE, et al: Prevalence and identification of abnormal lipoprotein levels in a biracial population aged 23 to 35 years (the CARDIA study). *Am J Cardiol* 1996;78:304-308.

14. Srinivasan SR, Segrest JP, Elkasabany AM, et al: Distribution and correlates of lipoproteins and their subclasses in black and white young adults. The Bogalusa Heart Study. *Atherosclerosis* 2001;159: 391-397.

15. Tyroler HAS, Glueck CJ, Christensen B, et al: Plasma high-density lipoprotein cholesterol comparisons in black and white populations. The Lipid Research Clinics Program Prevalence Study. *Circulation* 1980 62:IV99-IV107.

16. Anuurad E, Chiem A, Pearson TA, et al: Metabolic syndrome components in African-Americans and European-American patients and its relation to coronary artery disease. *Am J Cardiol* 2007;100: 839-834.

17. Zhu S, Heymsfield SB, Toyoshima H, et al: Race-ethnicity-specific waist circumference cutoffs for identifying cardiovascular disease risk factors. *Am J Clin Nutr* 2005;81:409-415.

18. Sharma S, Malarcher AM, Giles WH, et al: Racial, ethnic and socioeconomic disparities in the clustering of cardiovascular disease risk factors. *Ethnic Dis* 2004;14:43-48.

19. Winkleby MA, Kraemer HC, Ahn DK, et al: Ethnic and socioeconomic differences in cardiovascular disease risk factors: findings for women from the Third National Health and Nutrition Examination Survey, 1988-1994. *JAMA* 1998;280:356-362.

20. Gaillard TR, Schuster DP, Bossetti BM, et al: The impact of socioeconomic status on cardiovascular risk factors in African-Americans at high risk for type II diabetes. *Diabetes Care* 1997;20:745-752.

21. Signorello LB, Schlundt DG, Cohen SS, et al: Comparing diabetes prevalence between African Americans and Whites of similar socioeconomic status. *Am J Public Health* 2007;97:2260-2267.

22. Ranjit N, Diez-Roux AV, Shea S, et al: socioeconomic position, race/ethnicity, and inflammation in the Multi-Ethnic Study of Atherosclerosis. *Circulation* 2007;116:2383-2390.

23. Alley DE, Seeman TE, Ki Kim J, et al: Socioeconomic status and C-reactive protein levels in the US population: NHANES IV. *Brain Behav Immun* 2006;20:494-504.

24. Becker DM, Yanek LR, Johnson WR Jr, et al: Impact of a community-based multiple risk factor intervention on cardiovascular risk in black families with a history of premature coronary disease. *Circulation* 2005;111:1298-1304.

Chapter 2

Prevention of Cardiovascular Disease in Women

L. Veronica Lee, MD, and JoAnne Micale Foody, MD

The death rate for women from a cardiovascular event—such as myocardial infarction (MI), hypertensive heart disease, or stroke—is approximately 245 in 1,000, which is 10-fold the death rate that women have for breast cancer.[1] Although recent reductions in overall death rates from cardiovascular disease (CVD) have exceeded the American Heart Association (AHA) goals of a 25% reduction in CVD and stroke, declines in mortality have been significantly less in women. In women, more than one third of all deaths result from heart disease and in the United States, most heart disease deaths are in women (52.8%, 459,096 in 2004), not men. Although women have often erroneously been described as being "protected" from heart disease, and although the presentation of heart disease in women lags behind men by 10 years, we now know that heart disease is not only a disease of men or older women. In fact, heart disease is the second leading cause of death in women 45 to 64 years of age and the third leading cause of death in women 25 to 44 years of age.[2] Despite these compelling statistics, a survey by the AHA demonstrated that only 57% of women were aware that heart disease poses a significant risk factor for death in women. Unfortunately, heart disease continues to be viewed by health professionals and patients alike as a disease that primarily affects middle-aged men.

Much of the gender disparity in CVD may relate to the significant differences between the sexes in cardiovascular risk factors. In fact, modification of risk factors and how they affect disease are different between men and women. A recent analysis of the National Health and Nutrition Examination Survey (NHANES) attributes 47% of the decrease in cardiovascular death over the past 2 decades to improvement in treatment, including not only acute therapies and revascularization, but also primary and secondary prevention.[3] In this assessment, at least 44% of the decrease was due to risk factor reduction. This chapter reviews current data about the unique sex-specific characteristics of risk for CVD and examines the current knowledge of ways to improve clinical outcomes by reducing key risk factors for CVD.

Risk Factors of Cardiovascular Disease

While the traditional risk factors for CVD are not different for men and women, their impact on men and women vary greatly. The high rate of coronary artery disease (CAD) in women is in part because of the increase in significant risk factors. In general, women have a higher prevalence of all traditional risk factors compared to men, with the exception of tobacco use. Of women 20 years of age or older, a third have hypertension, nearly half have a total cholesterol of ≥200 mg/dL, nearly a quarter have prediabetes, almost one fifth smoke cigarettes, more than one third are obese with a body mass index (BMI) ≥30, and more than two thirds report a sedentary lifestyle.[3] With the exception of smoking, these risk factors are increasing and associated with the obesity epidemic.

Hypertension

Hypertension is the most common of CVD risk factor for women, with 85% of all women in the US being hypertensive by 75 years of age. Women tend to develop hypertension later as they transition into menopause and tend to develop primarily systolic hypertension rather than diastolic hypertension. Other hemodynamic parameters are also different between the sexes, with women having a higher cardiac output, lower systemic vascular resistance, and wider pulse pressure.[4] Before menopause, risk factors for the development of hypertension in women include secondary causes of hypertension, renal arterial stenosis, oral contraceptive use, and pregnancy.

During and after menopause, the development of hypertension in women is independent of BMI and age, both known risk factors of hypertension (for either gender), but is related to menopause.[5] The mechanism for development of hypertension in menopausal women is believed to be the lack of estrogen, resulting in vasoconstriction from both renin-angiotensin-aldosterone and sodium-sensitive pathways.[6,7] Potentially treatable contributing factors include folate deficiency, loss of the nocturnal dip, and sleep apnea. Dietary supplementation with folic acid has been shown to decrease the rate of new onset hypertension in women.[8] The nocturnal dip (10 mm Hg decrease in systolic blood pressure [SBP]) normally seen during sleep is lost when a woman enters menopause and can be restored with hormonal therapy.[9] Loss of the nocturnal dip has been associated with an increase risk of cardiovascular events.

Women do benefit from therapy for hypertension, although in a meta-analysis of seven trials that demonstrated this benefit, it was less pronounced in women than in men, who experienced a lower cardiovascular event rate.[10] In the Sibrafiban Versus Aspirin to Yield Maximum Protection from Ischemic Heart Events Post-Acute Coronary Syndromes (SYMPHONY) trial, hypertensive women with an acute coronary syndrome (ACS) were given more medications than men, but achieved target blood pressure control less often. We now have many choices for anti-hypertensive therapy, including angiotensin-converting enzyme (ACE) inhibitors, angiotensin receptor blockers (ARBs), β-blockers, calcium channel blockers (CCBs), and diuretics. Women appear to respond similarly as men to these blood pressure-lowering agents; however, women report more side effects than do men. This becomes an important consideration when prescribing medications for women with respect to improving compliance. On average, for men and women, it will take more than two medications to achieve a goal of a blood pressure <140/90 mm Hg, and combining two blood pressure medications into one pill has been shown to improve compliance. Given that women start with a lower blood pressure than men in their early adulthood, perhaps a lower target blood pressure is indicated for women than men. In view of this, the recent AHA prevention guidelines emphasize the importance of maintaining an optimal blood pressure <120 mm Hg for women.

There are limited data for therapy in women with chronic or new onset hypertension during pregnancy, although these are known to be significant risks for maternal and fetal mortality, premature delivery, abruptio placentae, thromboembolism, and hemorrhage. Frequently, therapy is withheld until SBP is >160 mm Hg or diastolic blood pressure (DBP) is >105 mm Hg. We know that hypertension during pregnancy is associated with the development of maternal vascular complications, such as eclampsia, subsequently increases the risk of developing long-term hypertension, and increases cardiovascular risk. Current recommended therapies during pregnancy include methyldopa, labetalol, hydralazine, nifedipine, and nicardipine.

Dyslipidemia

Low levels of high-density lipoprotein cholesterol (HDL-C) and high levels of low-density lipoprotein cholesterol (LDL-C) have been shown to be independent risk factors for CAD for both men and women. Although concentrations can vary with genetics, age, physical activity, and diet for both sexes, lipoprotein levels and, consequently, CAD risk, have been shown to vary with ovarian function. Women's total cholesterol levels increase at a slower rate than men's until the sixth decade, when they rapidly increase and then exceed age-matched men. For a given concentration of total cholesterol, women have a lower risk of CAD as compared to men. This is supported by the Framingham investigators, who demonstrated that at total cholesterol levels above 295 mg/dL, the rate of MI in women was 60% that in men.[11]

High-Density Lipoprotein Cholesterol. High-density lipoprotein cholesterol concentrations also change with age, with boys initially having higher levels than girls until puberty. During puberty, the HDL-C levels decline in boys and stay the same for girls. After puberty, HDL-C levels do not change in men while the levels slowly increase in women, until menopause, when they are about 20% higher in women than in men. After menopause, HDL-C levels decline by about 3.5 mg/dL, rising to a higher level in women than in men through old age.[12] Higher concentrations of HDL-C have been shown to be protective against developing CAD for both sexes. However, this effect is more pronounced in women, as demonstrated by the Framingham study, which found that every 10 mg/dL increase in HDL-C reduced the risk of CAD by 40% to 50%. That study concluded that this translated to HDL offsetting the atherogenic effect of LDL-C by 2-fold. Even at levels of HDL-C between 35 mg/dL and 50 mg/dL, increases in both CAD and CAD-related mortality have been documented. This has resulted in the current recommendations by the American College of Cardiology (ACC) for a higher HDL-C target concentration in women.[13]

Low-Density Lipoprotein Cholesterol. Although women have lower concentrations of LDL-C than do men from birth, menopause increases those concentrations after the middle of the fifth decade. During menopause, LDL levels rise abruptly, but remain unchanged in age-matched men.

Postmenopausal women generally have higher LDL levels than men.[14] Although independent of HDL, an LDL level of 130 mg/dL or higher has been established for men and women as a risk factor for CAD, but there is controversy about the role of LDL as a risk factor in women. In the limited prospective studies available for LDL levels and CAD risk in women, a very high LDL concentration carries the same poor prognosis for both men and women. However, mild elevations of LDL have not been found to be associated with the same degree of risk in women as compared to men, possibly because of the cardioprotective effects of the generally higher concentrations of HDL in women. The recently published Primary Prevention of Cardiovascular Disease with Pravastatin in Japan (MEGA) study is a prospective, randomized, open-label study of Japanese women and men 40 to 70 years of age with total cholesterol of 5.7 to 7.0 mmol/L receiving either 10 or 20 mg/d of pravastatin or dietary counseling.[15] Of the subjects enrolled, 68.4% were women (n= 5,356) and the incidence of CVD was lower in women than men by 2 to 3 times. Cardiovascular disease events (sudden death, fatal or non-fatal MI, angina, and revascularization) were 26% lower in treated women (19.1% lower cholesterol than baseline) than in those with only dietary counseling (4.9% lower cholesterol) (P=NS). These were comparable reductions to those observed in men. Treatment with pravastatin in women 60 years of age or older demonstrated a greater benefit than in younger women. In younger women with isolated elevations of LDL-C, additional risks such as diabetes, hormonal status, and family history should be considered before initiating medical therapy, but dietary counseling should continue to be given to all as an important lifestyle modification.

Triglycerides

Triglycerides (Tg) increase with age for both men and women, with women having a slower rate of increase. In middle-age men, Tg levels start to decline, while Tg levels in women continue to increase until 70 years of age, when women and men have equal mean levels of Tg. Triglyceride levels, when adjusted for multiple risk factors, are independent predictors of CAD risk. In older postmenopausal women, elevated Tg levels are common and may be the result of comorbid conditions such as the presence of atherogenic lipoproteins, obesity, metabolic syndrome, and insulin resistance.

Diabetes Mellitus

Irrespective of age, diabetes mellitus is one of the most significant risk factors for the development of CAD in women, doubling the risk for MI and tripling the incidence of CAD compared to nondiabetic women. In comparison, diabetic men have only twice the incidence of CAD compared to nondiabetic men. Gender-related differences in the age of onset of cardiovascular morbidity and mortality is lost in diabetic women. Part of the reason for the higher risk seen in diabetic women may be that many have multiple risk factors, such as smoking, obesity, and hypertension.

Diabetic women frequently have multiple cardiovascular risk factors that have been identified as part of the metabolic syndrome: elevated SBP, low HDL levels, high Tg levels, increased BMI, and impaired glucose tolerance. As a whole, diabetic women as compared to nondiabetic women have higher lipoprotein levels more dramatically elevated than diabetic and nondiabetic men.[16] In a recent study of diabetics with a history of CAD, women had less controlled SBP (46.6% vs 41.2%) and LDL-C (28.3% vs 22.4%) than did men without significant differences in intensity of medical regimens.[14] This suggests that there may be a clustering of risk factors contributing to the increased CVD event rate seen in diabetics. A recent study assessing the association of risk factors with CVD over years of follow-up demonstrated the highest hazard ratios (HR) for diabetes (5.38) and smoking (3.84) in the first 10

35

years in women, declining over time to the lowest point at >20 years of follow-up (1.71 and 1.60, respectively). Body mass index had a higher HR for men during the first 10 years, and no significant association was found to change over time with other risk factors.[17]

Smoking

Since 1965 there has been a 50% decline in smoking in people over 18 years of age.[18] As of 2005, however, 23.9% of men and 18.1% of women continue to smoke in the US. Women smokers die 14.5 years earlier and men smokers 13.2 years earlier than do nonsmokers. The incidence of MI is dose–dependent in women who smoke over the age of 44, increasing from 2.5% for those smoking 1-5 cigarettes daily to 74.6% for those smoking more than 40 cigarettes daily.[19] Smoking is also known to increase the risk of stroke, peripheral arterial disease, and aortic aneurysm, to alter cholesterol levels, elevate blood pressure, cause endothelial dysfunction, and increase restenosis in cardiovascular stents. Smoking has declined in men more rapidly than in women, but there is a higher prevalence of smoking among young women than in young men 17 years old or younger. The reasons for starting and continuing to smoke are different for women and men, making smoking a distinctive behavioral risk factor between the sexes.

Obesity and Physical Inactivity

Obesity is an independent risk factor for the development of CAD in women, as shown in the Framingham study in patients who were followed for 26 years. In this study, CAD was seen at increased rates in middle-aged women with only mild to moderate increases in weight, while obese women had an increase of 30% to 40% of CAD presentations.[20] A similar age-adjusted relative risk of CAD was demonstrated in the Nurses' Health Study in women with a BMI of 25 to 29 kg/m^2 as compared to a BMI of >29 kg/m^2, which showed an increase in relative risk from 1.8 to 3.3, respectively.[21]

In 2005, 33.2% of women in the US more than 20 years of age had BMIs of 25 or higher, and are at an increased risk of developing CAD.[3]

In both men and women, the waist-to-hip ratio as a measure of distribution of body fat may be more important than absolute weight measurements for determining increases in CVD risk. An excessive waist-to-hip ratio is called truncal obesity (the apple or android, male pattern, instead of the pear or female pattern) and is associated with lower HDL and higher LDL concentrations and, in women, with a significant increase in CAD.

Sleep apnea, commonly associated with obesity, is a significant, independent risk factor for CVD and arrhythmia and is thought to be less prevalent in women, according to epidemiologic, clinic-based studies. But sleep apnea may be underdiagnosed because of gender-specific differences in presentation and because health professionals often are not aware of these differences in women.[22] As in CVD, women with sleep apnea present with more fatigue[23] and more frequent sleep disturbances, including difficulty falling and staying asleep.[24] Daytime sleepiness was reported more often in women in the Wisconsin Sleep Cohort Study, even in cases of little or no sleep apnea. Because sleep apnea is often undertreated in women, it is important to ask patients about snoring, fatigue, daytime sleepiness, and sleep habits. A potential mechanistic difference between men and women may exist, as suggested by a difference in the pattern of episodes of apnea and hypopnea, most occurring in rapid eye movement (REM) sleep in women and in non-REM sleep in men.[25,26]

Lack of exercise is now considered to be as much of a risk factor as smoking in the development of CAD.[27,28] In general, women engage in less vigorous exercise and lead a more sedentary lifestyle than do men. There was a modest 8.6% increase in physical activity in women from 2001 to 2005, defined as at least 30 minutes of physical activity on most days (46.7% of women did so in 2005).[29] Women who exercise have shown modest increases in fitness, when compared to women with a sedentary lifestyle, such as lower blood pressure, lower blood glucose levels, improved lipid profiles, and weight reduction.[30,31] Because of the importance of exercise in prevention programs, the AHA has stepped up efforts to encourage exercise in the workplace.

Prevention

While the Framingham risk score has been the mainstay to calculate risk, it has significant limitations in women and is likely to seriously underestimate risk in women. The Framingham risk score does not account for family history, obesity, or insulin resistance, all of which are important risk factors in women. As a result, the new ACC guidelines suggest that all women who have any risk factors for CAD are at risk and should be treated as such. These guidelines establish much lower levels of risk factors as optimal and are generally more aggressive than those of either the National Cholesterol Education Program Adult Treatment Panel III (NCEP ATP III) or the Seventh Report of the Joint National Committee on Prevention, Detection, Evaluation, and Treatment of High Blood Pressure (JNC 7). Optimal-risk women are defined as having a Framingham risk score of <10% and a healthy lifestyle with no other risk factors; high-risk patients include not only women with existing CVD, but also those with history of stroke, peripheral vascular disease, aortic aneurysm, chronic kidney disease (CKD), diabetes, and a 10-year Framingham global risk ≥20%. The at-risk category is reserved for all other women, emphasizing that most women have risk factors for CVD that need to be addressed by the health-care system.[20] Table 2-1 provides a summary of preventive care for nonpregnant women.

A woman's degree of risk should be identified and an individualized program adopted to address the key risk factors for her. Interventions should include lifestyle modifications, preventive therapy, and further diagnostic assessments. In addition to CAD prevention, risk for stroke and leading causes of stroke, such as atrial fibrillation, should be evaluated because stroke is associated with many of the same risk factors. Recent studies have also suggested an increased risk of developing cancer in patients with similar cardiovascular risk factors.

Hormone Replacement Therapy

Recent clinical trials have suggested that hormone replacement therapy (HRT) to treat menopause does not reduce risk for CAD and, moreover, is potentially harmful. The Women's Health Initiative (WHI) is a randomized, controlled trial of 16,605 healthy postmenopausal women treated with placebo or combined estrogen/progesterone therapy. Part of the study was stopped early because an increased risk of breast cancer was detected (HR, 1.26), as well as an increase risk of pulmonary embolism (HR, 2.13), stroke (HR 1.41), and cardiovascular events (HR, 1.29).[32,33] Similar results were found in a meta-analysis of 22 randomized trials (n=4,124), which found an increase in cardiovascular events in women treated with hormonal therapy as compared to placebo (HR, 1.39, 95% confidence interval [CI], 0.48–3.95).[34]

A multicenter, randomized, double-blind, placebo-controlled trial of 2,763 postmenopausal women, the Heart and Estrogen/progestin Replacement Study (HERS), was the first to study the possible cardioprotective effects of estrogen.[35] In the first year, there was a 52% increased risk of cardiovascular events in women receiving HRT. Even after a 6.8-year follow-up, no evidence of cardiovascular benefit was detected.[36] Additional studies have not demonstrated benefit in reducing the end points of cardiac death, MI, or progression of CAD, even in the setting of significantly improved LDL and HDL. These studies include the Estrogen in the Prevention of Reinfarction Trial (ESPRIT) (n=1,017, 2-year therapy), the Estrogen Replacement and Atherosclerosis (ERA) trial (n=309, 3.2- year follow-up),

Table 2-1: ABCDEs for CVD Prevention in Nonpregnant Women

A	Angiotensin-converting enzyme (ACE) inhibitors	For women post-MI, women with CHF, LV systolic dysfunction, LV hypertrophy (LVH), nephropathy, CVD, and/or diabetes or hypertension. Similar recommendations for men. Avoid in pregnancy. Increased incidence of side effects compared to men (cough, angioedema).
	Angiotensin II receptor blockers (ARBs)	Women with diabetes, nephropathy, hypertension, or LVH. For women who are ACE inhibitor intolerant, or have post-MI, CHF, LV systolic dysfunction. Similar recommendations for men. Avoid in pregnancy.
	Antianginals	Women with known inducible ischemia and nitrate responsive chest pain without significant CAD. Include nitrates, CCBs, and β-blockers.
	Anticoagulants: warfarin, heparin, GP IIb/IIIa platelet receptor inhibitors	Warfarin: women with atrial fibrillation, LV aneurysm, or LV thrombus. Heparin (UF or LMWH): Modify dosing per weight as in men. GP IIb/IIIa receptor inhibitors: Women at high risk (troponin-positive NSTEMI), may have increased risk of bleeding. Not for troponin-negative NSTEMI.

CHF=congestive heart failure, DM=diabetes mellitus, LV=left ventricular, NSTEMI=non-ST segment myocardial infarction

A	Antiplatelet: aspirin, clopidogrel	For women at risk of stroke, or age >65 without contraindications. Women with known CVD or at high risk. Clopidogrel in same patients if aspirin intolerant or in women after stent for CVD.
B	β-blockers	Women post-MI, at high risk of MI, inducible ischemia, symptomatic tachycardias, CHF, and hypertension.
	Blood pressure control	Women with low CVD risk <140/90 mm Hg. Women at high risk CVD, CVD, DM, nephropathy <130/80 mm Hg. Therapy should be risk directed (eg, β-blockers post-MI); otherwise, consider ACE inhibitors, CCBs, and thiazide diruetics. Second tier: ARBs and β-blockers. Consider secondary causes of hypertension (renal arterial stenosis), sleep apnea, lifestyle modification: low sodium, high potassium (unless kidney disease) diet, folic acid supplementation, exercise, stress management, smoking cessation.
C	Calcium channel blockers (CCBs)	

(continued on next page)

Table 2-1: ABCDEs for CVD Prevention in Nonpregnant Women *(continued)*

C	Cigarette smoking	Smoke-out date, counseling, bupropion, nicotine patch, varenicline. Weight gain associated with cessation normalizes within 1 year if related to smoking cessation.
	Cholesterol	Goal: HDL >50 mg/dL, increase exercise, 3 oz red wine/day, weight loss, fish or flaxseed oil, niacin, fibrates. Goal: LDL <100 mg/dL for high risk, consider lowering to <70 mg/dL, diet, weight loss, exercise, HMG CoA reductase inhibitors (statins), niacin, fibrates, increased fiber in diet, avoid *trans* fatty acids (hydrogenated or partially hydrogenated oils). Goal: Tg <150 mg/dL, improve glycemic control, improve diet (less processed food), weight loss, exercise.
D	Depression and anxiety	Women should be screened and treated for depression and anxiety, since both can increase the risk of CVD and make risk factors harder to treat.

D	Diabetes	Impaired fasting glucose (>110-124 mg/dL): lifestyle change, weight loss, exercise. Diabetes: improve glycemic control with lifestyle changes, medications with goal of HbA_{1c} <6.5%. Lowest risk at HbA_{1c} <6%.
	Diet and weight management, sleep apnea	Emphasis on lifestyle change, portion control, and a diet high in fiber, fruits, vegetables, whole grains, low in sodium, low in saturated fat and cholesterol, avoid processed foods, BMI <25, waist-to-hip ratio ≤0.8, body fat of <25% (most accurate measure). Screen women for sleep apnea if snoring, sleep disturbance, hypertension, fatigue, weight gain, atypical chest pain, arrhythmia, CVD, or stroke. Not all patients are overweight.
	Diuretics, direct renin inhibitors	Caution in women with symptoms of dehydration, dryness, and incontinence. Excellent at lower dose as adjunctive therapy for hypertension. Direct renin inhibitors have few side effects in women, but clinical outcome trial data are pending.

(continued on next page)

Table 2-1: ABCDEs for CVD Prevention in Nonpregnant Women *(continued)*

E	Ejection fraction	ACE inhibitor (ARB if intolerant) and β-blocker for all women with CHF or decreased LV systolic function. Aldosterone antagonist if severe CHF and low-risk hyperkalemia. Use digoxin with caution. High-risk women may be candidates for ICD; apply same guidelines as in men.
	Exercise	Aerobic exercise at least 30 min/day on most days. For women doing little or no exercise, initiate a walking regimen with goals using a pedometer. For weight loss, may need to increase to an hour. Resistance training with lighter weights and frequent repetitions. Address limitations to physical exercise with physical therapy. Cardiac rehabilitation for women post-MI, revascularization, CHF, chronic angina.
	Ego and self-esteem	Women as primary caregivers often put their needs last, and this social view has to be addressed when prescribing therapy and treatment.

ICD=implantable cardiac defibrillator

and the Women's Angiographic Vitamin and Estrogen (WAVE) trial (n=423).[37,38] Secondary prevention of stroke has also not been shown to benefit from estrogen therapy.[39,40]

These findings oppose the epidemiologic and pathophysiologic data that suggest that estrogen replacement is beneficial. It is well known that estrogen therapy improves lipid profile by raising HDL and lowering LDL. In addition, HRT has been shown to slow the progression of carotid intimal thickness and have impressive effects on diastolic measures of heart function.[41,42] Beneficial effects from HRT have also been observed on 24-hour blood pressure monitoring in menopausal women.[43] It is unclear if another method of delivery, or another combination of HRT, would result in benefit, or if the use of HRT in younger women in early menopause as opposed to much older women years after menopause would affect cardiovascular outcomes. However, given the wealth of data from clinical trials, long-term HRT cannot be recommended for prevention of CAD. The AHA states that the initiation of HRT in women with CAD for prevention of cardiovascular events cannot be supported by current data. A decision to initiate or continue HRT in the setting of known or absent CAD must be made weighing the risks and non-CAD benefits to the patient.[44]

We await the results of studies such as the Kronos Early Estrogen Prevention Study (KEEPS) to inform clinical decision making.

References

1.   National Center for Health Statistics: Center for Disease Control and Prevention. Compressed mortality file: underlying cause of death 1979-2004. Atlanta GA. Centers for Disease Control and Prevention. Available at http://wonder.cdc.gov/mortSQL.html. Accessed January 2008.

2.   Rosamond W, Flegal K, Furie K, et al: Heart disease and stroke statistics—2008 update: a report from the American Heart Association Statistics Committee and Stroke Statistics Subcommittee. *Circulation* 2008;117:e25-146.

3.   Ford ES, Ajani UA, Croft JB, et al: Explaining the decrease in U.S. deaths from coronary disease, 1980–2000. *N Engl J Med* 2007;356:2388-2398.

4.   Safar ME, Smulyan H: Hypertension in women. *Am J Hypertens* 2004;17(1):82-87.

5.   Zanchetti A, Facchetti R, Cesana GC, et al: Menopause-related blood pressure increase and its relationship to age and body mass index: the SIMONA epidemiological study. *J Hypertens* 2005;23:2269-2276.

6.   Ramírez-Exposito MJ, Martínez-Martos JM: Hypertension, RAS, and gender: what is the role of aminopeptidases? *Heart Fail Rev* 2008;13:355-365.

7.   Schulman IH, Raij L: Salt sensitivity and hypertension after menopause: role of nitric oxide and angiotensin II. *Am J Nephrol* 2006;26:170-180.

8.   Forman JP, Rimm EB, Stampfer MJ et al: Folate intake and the risk of incident hypertension among US women. *JAMA* 2005; 293(3):320-329.

9.   Butkevich A, Abraham C, Phillips RA: Hormone replacement therapy and 24-hour blood pressure profile of postmenopausal women. *Am J Hypertens* 2000;13:1039-1041.

10.   Gueyffier F, Boutitie F, Boissel JP: Effect of antihypertensive drug treatment on cardiovascular outcomes in women and men. A meta-analysis of individual patient data from randomized, controlled trials. The INDANA Investigators. *Ann Intern Med* 1997;126(10):761-767.

11.   Kannel WB: The Framingham Study: historical insight on the impact of cardiovascular risk factors in men versus women. *J Gend Specif Med* 2002;5:27-37.

12.   Bittner V: Lipoprotein abnormalities related to women's health. *Am J Cardiol* 2002;90:77i-84i.

13.   Mosca L. Banka CL, Benjamin EJ: Evidence-based guidelines for cardiovascular disease prevention in women: 2007 update. *Circulation* 2007;115:1-20.

14.   Ferrare A, Mangione CM, Kim C: Sex disparities in control and treatment of modifiable cardiovascular disease risk factors among patients with diabetes. *Diabetes Care* 2008;31:69-74.

15.   Mizuno K, Nakaya N, Ohashi Y, et al, on behalf of the MEGA Study Group: Usefulness of pravastatin in primary prevention of

cardiovascular events in women: analysis of the Management of Elevated cholesterol in the primary prevention Group of Adult Japanese (MEGA Study). *Circulation* 2008;117:494-502.

16. Walden CE, Knopp RH, Wahl PW, et al: Sex differences in the effect of diabetes mellitus on lipoprotein triglyceride and cholesterol concentrations. *N Engl J Med* 1984;311:953-959.

17. Berry JD, Dyer A, Carnethon M, et al: Association of traditional risk factors with cardiovascular death across 0 to 10, 10 to 20, and >20 years follow-up in men and women. *Am J Cardiol* 2008;101(1): 89-94.

18. National Center for Health Statistics: Health, United States, 2007: with chartbook on trends in the health of Americans. Hyattsville, Md: National Center for Health Statistics; 2007. Available at: http://www.cdc.gov/nchs/hus.htm. Accessed January 2008.

19. US Department of Health & Human Services: The health consequences of smoking: a report of the surgeon general. Atlanta, Ga: US Department of Health & Human Services, Public Health Service, Centers for Disease Control and Prevention, National Center for Chronic Disease Prevention and Health Promotion, Office on Smoking and Health; 2004. Available at: www.cdc.gov/tobacco/sgr/sgr_2004/index.htm. Accessed January 2008.

20. Mosca L, Grundy SM, Judelson D, et al: Guide to preventive cardiology for women. AHA/ACC Scientific Statement Consensus panel statement. *Circulation* 1999;99:2480-2484.

21. Kritz-Silverstein D, Barrett-Connor E: Long-term postmenopausal hormone use, obesity, and fat distribution in older women. *JAMA* 1996;275:46-49.

22. Young T: Analytic epidemiology studies of sleep disordered breathing—what explains the gender difference in sleep disordered breathing. *Sleep* 1993;16(suppl 8):S1-S2.

23. Chervin RD: Sleepiness, fatigue, tiredness, and lack of energy in obstructive sleep apnea. *Chest* 2000;118(2):372-379.

24. Baldwin CM, Griffith KA, Nieto FJ, et al: The association of sleep-disordered breathing and sleep symptoms with quality of life in the Sleep Heart Health Study. *Sleep* 2001;24(1):96-105.

25. Ware JC, McBrayer RH, Scott JA: Influence of sex and age on duration and frequency of sleep apnea events. *Sleep* 2000;23(2): 165-170.

26. O'Connor C, Thornley KS, Hanly PJ: Gender differences in the polysomnographic features of obstructive sleep apnea. *Am J Respir Crit Care Med* 2000;161:1465-1472.

27. Dubbert PM, Carithers T, Sumner AE, et al: Obesity, physical inactivity, and risk for cardiovascular disease. *Am J Med Sci* 2002; 324:116-126.

28. Lawler JM, Hu Z, Green JS, et al: Combination of estrogen replacement and exercise protects against HDL oxidation in post-menopausal women. *Int J Sports Med* 2002;23:477-483.

29. Centers for Disease Control and Prevention: 2001 and 2005 BRFSS summary data quality reports. Atlanta, GA: US Department of Health & Human Services, CDC; 2002 and 2006. Available at http://ftp.cdc.gov/pub/data/brfss/2001summarydataqualityreport.pdf and http://ftp.cdc.gov/pub/data/brfss/2005summarydataqualityreport. pdf. Accessed January 2008.

30. Miller TD, Fletcher GF: Exercise and coronary artery disease prevention. *Cardiologia* 1998;43:43-51.

31. Grundy SM, Bazzarre T, Cleeman J, et al: Prevention Conference V: Beyond secondary prevention: identifying the high-risk patient for primary prevention: medical office assessment: Writing Group I. *Circulation* 2000;101:E3-E11.

32. Rossouw JE, Anderson GL, Prentice RL, et al: Risks and benefits of estrogen plus progestin in healthy postmenopausal women: principal results from the Women's Health Initiative randomized controlled trial. *JAMA* 2002;288:321-333.

33. Hays J, Ockene JK, Brunner RL, et al: Effects of estrogen plus progestin on health-related quality of life. *N Engl J Med* 2003;348:1839-1854.

34. Hemminki E, McPherson K: Impact of postmenopausal hormone therapy on cardiovascular events and cancer: pooled data from clinical trials. *BMJ* 1997;315:149-153.

35. Grady D, Applegate W, Bush T, et al: Heart and Estrogen/progestin Replacement Study (HERS): design, methods, and baseline characteristics. *Control Clin Trials* 1998;19:314-335.

36. Grady D, Herrington D, Bittner V, et al: Cardiovascular disease outcomes during 6.8 years of hormone therapy: Heart and Estrogen/progestin Replacement Study follow-up (HERS II). *JAMA* 2002;288:49-57. (Erratum, *JAMA* 2002;288:1064.)

37. Cherry N, Gilmour K, Hannaford P: Oestrogen therapy for prevention of reinfarction in postmenopausal women: a randomized placebo controlled trial. *Lancet* 2002;360:2001.

38. Herrington DM, Howard TD, Hawkins GA, et al: Estrogen-receptor polymorphisms and effects of estrogen replacement on high-density lipoprotein cholesterol in women with coronary disease. *N Engl J Med* 2002;346:967-974.

39. Hurn PD, Brass LM: Estrogen and stroke: a balanced analysis. *Stroke* 2003;34:338-341.

40. Viscoli CM, Brass LM, Kernan WN, et al: A clinical trial of estrogen-replacement therapy after ischemic stroke. *N Engl J Med* 2001;345:1243-1249.

41. Dubuisson JT, Wagenknecht LE, D'Agostino RB: Association of hormone replacement therapy and carotid wall thickness in women with and without diabetes. *Diabetes Care* 1998;21(11):1790-1796.

42. Aldrighi JM, Alecrin IN, Caldas MA, et al: Effects of estradiol on myocardial global performance index in hypertensive postmenopausal women. *Gynecol Endocrinol* 2004;19(5):282-292.

43. Kaya C, Dincer Cengiz S, Cengiz B, et al: The long-term effects of low-dose 17β-estradiol and dydrogesterone hormone replacement therapy on 24-h ambulatory blood pressure in hypertensive postmenopausal women: a 1-year randomized, prospective study. *Climacteric* 2006;9(6):437-445.

44. Mosca L, Collins P, Herrington DM, et al: Hormone replacement therapy and cardiovascular disease: a statement for healthcare professionals from the American Heart Association. *Circulation* 2001;104:499-503.

Chapter 3

Risk Factors in Special Populations

By C. Tissa Kappagoda, MD, PhD,
and Ezra A. Amsterdam, MD

The Framingham Study was a landmark epidemiologic undertaking initiated in the United States in 1948 to determine the risk factors for the development of coronary heart disease (CHD) risk.[1] It eventually yielded gender-specific equations[2] to predict, "hard coronary heart disease risk according to age; diabetes (two casual blood sugar determinations >150 mg/dL or a single fasting value >140 mg/dL); smoking (regular smoking over the previous 12 months); blood pressure (as defined by Joint National Committee on Prevention, Detection, Evaluation, and Treatment of High Blood Pressure [JNC])[3]; and total, high-density lipoprotein (HDL), low-density lipoprotein (LDL), and very-low-density lipoprotein (VLDL) cholesterol." This concept was incorporated later into the recommendations of the Third Report of the National Cholesterol Education Program Expert Panel on Detection, Evaluation and Treatment of High Blood Cholesterol in Adults (Adult Treatment Panel III) (NCEP–ATP III) for assessment of global risk for CHD and its management in men and women.[4] These gender-specific predictive algorithms in asymptomatic individuals afforded scores (Framingham Risk Score [FRS]), which provided a 10-year global risk of developing CHD (Figures 3-1A and 3-1B). The risk, which is expressed as a percentage, has three levels: low: <10%; intermediate: 10% to 20%; and high >20%, and is calculated from gender, age, total cholesterol, HDL cholesterol, smoking, and blood pressure (with or without therapy). LDL cholesterol was a therapeutic target,[4,5] and not considered in the calculation of risk. Additionally, diabetes was considered a CHD equivalent, rather than a risk factor, with the same therapeutic targets as established vascular disease. The metabolic syndrome was considered a high-risk state, meriting aggressive management of lipids but was not specifically designated as a CHD equivalent.[4,5] The metabolic syndrome was defined by the NCEP III as a condition based on the presence of at least three of the following: abdominal obesity, elevated serum triglycerides (Tg), low serum HDL concentration, hypertension, and elevated blood glucose (>105 mg/dL). In the most recent modification of ATP III, an additional "very high risk" category was introduced, which included people with acute coronary syndromes and both CHD and diabetes.[5]

Several national forums in other countries have also adopted a similar approach and developed their own predictive algorithms.[6-10] Aside from minor modifications, such as those induced by the influence of socioeconomic factors[9] and geographic locations of subjects,[7] all these studies have supported the basic concept behind the Framingham Study.

The INTERHEART study[11] by Yusuf et al effectively "internationalized" the concept of global risk. It was a standardized case-control study of acute myocardial infarction (MI) undertaken in 52 countries drawn from every inhabited continent; 15,152 cases and 14,820 controls were enrolled to establish whether or not the risk factors for CHD had universal application. This study indicated that, worldwide, abnormal lipids, smoking, hypertension, diabetes, abdominal obesity, psychosocial factors, consumption of fruit and vegetables, alcohol consumption in moderation (these two are inverse risk factors), and lack of physical

Men

Age, yr	Points	Age, yr	Points
20-34	-9	55-59	8
35-39	-4	60-64	10
40-44	0	65-69	11
45-49	3	70-74	12
50-54	6	75-79	13

Total Cholesterol, mg/dL	Points				
	Age 20-39 yr	Age 40-49 yr	Age 50-59 yr	Age 60-69 yr	Age 70-79 yr
<160	0	0	0	0	0
160-199	4	3	2	1	0
200-239	7	5	3	1	0
240-279	9	6	4	2	1
≥280	11	8	5	3	1

	Points				
	Age 20-39 yr	Age 40-49 yr	Age 50-59 yr	Age 60-69 yr	Age 70-79 yr
Nonsmoker	0	0	0	0	0
Smoker	8	5	3	1	1

Figures 3-1A and B: Framingham risk-scoring table for calculating the 10-year risk for developing coronary heart disease (CHD). **3-1A:** Men; **3-1B:** Women. The risk factors include age, total cholesterol, HDL cholesterol, systolic blood pressure,

HDL, mg/dL	Points
≥60	-1
50-59	0
40-49	1
<40	2

Systolic BP, mm Hg	If Untreated	If Treated
<120	0	0
120-129	0	1
130-139	1	2
140-159	1	2
≥160	2	3

Point Total	10-Year Risk %	Point Total	10-Year Risk %
<0	<1	9	5
0	1	10	6
1	1	11	8
2	1	12	10
3	1	13	12
4	1	14	16
5	2	15	20
6	2	16	25
7	3	≥17	≥30
8	4		

treatment for hypertension, and cigarette smoking. Using the gender-specific table, the points for each risk factor are summed to yield the total score. The bottom part of each table gives the 10-year risk of developing CHD based on the total score.[2,4]

Women

Age, yr	Points	Age, yr	Points
20-34	-7	55-59	8
35-39	-3	60-64	10
40-44	0	65-69	12
45-49	3	70-74	14
50-54	6	75-79	16

Total Cholesterol, mg/dL	Points				
	Age 20-39 yr	Age 40-49 yr	Age 50-59 yr	Age 60-69 yr	Age 70-79 yr
<160	0	0	0	0	0
160-199	4	3	2	1	1
200-239	8	6	4	2	1
240-279	11	8	5	3	2
≥280	13	10	7	4	2

	Points				
	Age 20-39 yr	Age 40-49 yr	Age 50-59 yr	Age 60-69 yr	Age 70-79 yr
Nonsmoker	0	0	0	0	0
Smoker	8	5	3	1	1

Figures 3-1A and B: Framingham risk-scoring table for calculating the 10-year risk for developing coronary heart disease (CHD). **3-1A:** Men; **3-1B:** Women. The risk factors include age, total cholesterol, HDL cholesterol, systolic blood pressure,

HDL, mg/dL	Points
≥60	-1
50-59	0
40-49	1
<40	2

Systolic BP, mm Hg	If Untreated	If Treated
<120	0	0
120-129	1	3
130-139	2	4
140-159	3	5
≥160	4	6

Point Total	10-Year Risk %	Point Total	10-Year Risk %
<9	<1	18	5
9	1	19	8
10	1	20	11
11	1	21	14
12	1	22	17
13	2	23	22
14	2	24	27
15	3	≥25	≥30
16	4		
17	5		

treatment for hypertension, and cigarette smoking. Using the gender-specific table, the points for each risk factor are summed to yield the total score. The bottom part of each table gives the 10-year risk of developing CHD based on the total score.[2,4]

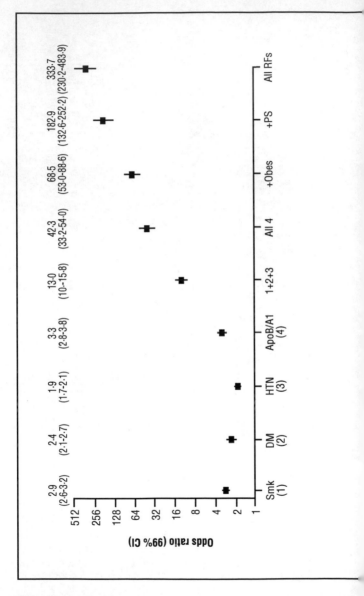

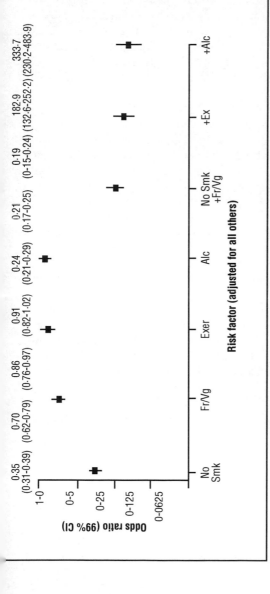

Figure 3-2: The effect of major risk factors for CHD on risk of a myocardial infarction (MI) from the INTERHEART study. Left: the effect of the presence of risk factors; Right: effect of the absence of risk factors or the presence of beneficial factors. Avoidance of smoking, daily consumption of fruit and vegetables, and regular physical activity significantly reduce the risk of MI (nearly 75% reduction in risk compared to a smoker with a poor lifestyle). A_{1c}=hemoglobin A_{1c}, Alc=alcohol consumption[11], ApoA1/Apo3=ratio of apolipoproteins, DM=diabetes, Fr/Vg=diet with adequate fruit and vegetables, HTN=hypertension, Obes=obesity, PS=psychosocial factors, Smk=smoking

activity accounted for 90% of the risk of MI in men and 94% in women (Figure 3-2). The study vindicated the use of the gender-specific algorithms for predicting CHD derived from the Framingham Study and helped put to rest the specious concept that only 50% of CHD could be accounted for by conventional risk factors (the "50% myth").

Risk Factors in African Americans

Although the rates of CHD have been declining for the past five decades in the US, the reduction in African Americans has been relatively small and, as a result, this group now has a disproportionate share of CHD burden in this country.[12]

Hypertension, Dyslipidemia, and Smoking

In the 1990s, the Atherosclerosis Risk in Communities (ARIC) Study[13] and the Jackson Heart Study (JHS)[14] were designed to explore the reasons for this trend. ARIC was a prospective study of cardiovascular disease in a cohort of 15,792 persons sampled from four US communities in 1987–1989. The cohort continues to be followed for morbidity and mortality. The ARIC study sample consisted at baseline of 45–to 64-year-old members of households in selected Minneapolis suburbs (Minnesota), Forsyth County (North Carolina), Washington County (Maryland), and Jackson (Mississippi), the latter sample from black residents only. There were three follow-up examinations over a median period of 10.2 years. The sample size was 14,054 (2,297 black women, 5,686 white women, 1,394 black men, 4,677 white men), and the number of incident CHD events was 1,064 (113, 232, 133, 586, respectively). Age-adjusted event rates were much higher for men than for women (data not shown). Black women had higher rates than white women ($P = 0.03$), and black men had lower rates than did white men ($P = 0.05$).

White women had statistically significantly larger hazard risk (HR) ratios related to total cholesterol than did

Table 3-1: Multivariable Adjusted Hazard Rate Ratios of CHD, by Sex and Race: the Atherosclerosis Risk in Communities Study, 1987–1998

	Women		Men	
Risk Factor	*Black*	*White*	*Black*	*White*
Systolic blood pressure (>20 mm Hg)	1.65	1.35	1.05	1.31
Total cholesterol (≤280 vs <200 mg/dL)	2.26	2.54	2.01	2.17
HDL (<35 vs ≤60 mg/dL)	2.92	3.35	2.21	3.37
Diabetes	1.86	2.95	1.6	1.19
Current Smoker	2.75	3.01	1.88	1.46

HDL=high-density lipoprotein

black women. White men had a larger HR ratio related to systolic blood pressure than did black men, but they had a smaller HR ratio related to antihypertensive medications, and white women had a smaller HR ratio related to systolic blood pressure than did black women (these comparisons statistically significant at $P < 0.05$ (Table 3-1 for details).[15]

In contrast, the JHS was initiated in 2000 as a single-site cohort study to identify the risk factors for the development of cardiovascular diseases in African Americans.[14] The cohort consisted of participants from the Jackson site of the ARIC Study and a sample of residents from the Jackson metropolitan area. There were approximately 6,500 men and women, 35-84 years of age, drawn from approximately 400 families. This study, while corroborating the findings of the ARIC study with respect to hypertension, also highlighted the prevalence of hypertension in African-American men and women, which was considerably more than that in Caucasians (Figure 3-3).

The participants in the Genetic Epidemiology Network of Arteriopathy (GENOA) study provided additional insights into the relationship between hypertension and serum lipids in African Americans. HDL-C levels were higher and triglyceride levels lower in African-American men and women than in their non-Hispanic white counterparts.[16] Despite this apparently favorable trend, LDL particle size (adjusted for CHD risk factors) was lower (P <0.0001) in African-American men and women than in their white counterparts even after adjustment for CHD risk factors, statin use, and estrogen use (in women), as well as physical activity and alcohol intake.[17] Additonally, in African Americans, elevated triglycerides were strongly predictive (≥150 mg/dL: 67% vs <150 mg/dL: 17%) of the presence of small, dense LDL particles (pattern B).[18] The clinical importance of a higher prevalence of small LDL particles remains controversial because their presence does not predict subclinical CHD in the form of coronary calcification.[19] Thus, further confirmatory studies are needed to establish whether lower LDL particle size contributes to higher risk of CHD in hypertensive African Americans.

Smoking is an important modifiable risk factor in all ethnic groups.[20] Despite efforts designed to discourage smoking, the number of active smokers has remained steady for several years. The Centers for Disease Control and Prevention (CDC) has reported that in the US slightly more than 20% of individuals between the ages of 18 and 64 smoke.[21] Among African Americans, the prevalence has remained steady at approximately 21%. The highest prevalence of smokers is among American Indians and Alaskan natives (32%).[21]

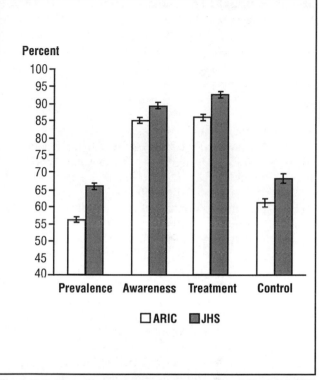

Figure 3-3: Hypertension status in Jackson Heart Study (JHS)[14] and Atherosclerosis Risk in Communities (ARIC) Study.[13] Error bars represent standard errors (SE). Hypertensive participants were classified into subgroups based on awareness, treatment, and control. Hypertension awareness was defined by a *yes* response to the questions: "Has your health-care provider ever told you that you have hypertension?" or "Were any of the medications you took in the past 2 weeks for high blood pressure?" Hypertension treatment was defined as currently taking 1 of 7 classes of antihypertensive medications. Hypertension was considered a new diagnosis for unaware and untreated participants with systolic blood pressure ≥140 mm Hg or diastolic blood pressure ≥90 mm Hg. Overall hypertension control was defined as blood pressure <140/90 mm Hg.

Obesity, Metabolic Syndrome, Diabetes, Peripheral Arterial Disease

Besides hypertension, hyperlipidemia, and smoking, the other important risk factors that merit discussion in African Americans are obesity, the metabolic syndrome, diabetes, and peripheral arterial disease (PAD). The presence of these factors places even asymptomatic individuals in a high risk category as defined by NCEP III.[4,5]

The National Health and Nutrition Examination Survey (NHANES) study (1999-2002) showed that prevalence of PAD was significantly higher in African Americans (7.8%) than in whites (3.4%) or in Mexican Americans (5.1%) (P <0.001).[22] African Americans had the highest rates of PAD despite similar control of conventional risk factors such as hypertension and hyperlipidemia between racial groups. However, African Americans had what was described as higher allostatic loads, which are a global marker of dysregulation of the inflammatory, metabolic, and cardiovascular systems. Similar data were found in subjects in the San Diego Population Study,[23] which evaluated 104 persons with PAD and 164 age- and gender-matched control subjects. Nine novel cardiovascular risk factors, which were considered components of the allostatic load, were measured: homocysteine, lipoprotein(a) [Lp(a)], C-reactive protein, fibrinogen, tumor necrosis factor-α, von Willebrand factor, prothrombin fragment 1-2, D-dimer, and plasmin antiplasmin. African Americans had 3-fold higher odds of PAD in age- and gender-matched models (odds ratio [OR] 3.1; P <0.01), an association that was modestly attenuated by adjustment for traditional (OR 2.4; P=0.06) and novel cardiovascular risk markers (OR 1.9; P=0.18). Among the novel factors, the attenuation was primarily associated with fibrinogen and lipoprotein(a). It was concluded that traditional and novel CVD risk factors only partially explained the higher prevalence of PAD in African Americans.

Risk Factors in Hispanic Populations
The Hispanic Paradox

It has been suggested that Hispanics have a lower all-cause and cardiovascular mortality than the general US population despite an increased prevalence of diabetes and obesity, lower socioeconomic status, and barriers to health care. This finding has been referred to as the Hispanic paradox, which has been extended to apply especially to individuals who have migrated to the US in good health from Latin American countries. A formal investigation of the Hispanic paradox[24] suggested that this phenomenon coincided with a change from the classification of deaths and population by Spanish surname to the use of "Hispanic-origin"-type questions in the census and vital statistics. From an evaluation of population statistics for Texas, it was concluded that there was no Hispanic paradox and that this finding was related to inconsistencies in counts of Hispanic-origin deaths and populations. A substantially similar conclusion was reached[25] from an analysis of 140 publications that addressed multiple aspects of CVD in US Hispanic and Latin American populations over a 30-year period. It concluded that "the lower mortality in Hispanics is not 'genuine,' but rather is caused by migratory demographic factors and probably mild distortions due to selection combined with mild reporting errors that may produce the appearance of a paradox when there is none at all." Such evidence that is available to support the idea of a paradox points to an effect attributable to acculturation (see Chapter 12).

Several studies have examined the prevalence of pre-clinical coronary artery disease (CAD) in the form of coronary artery calcification in Hispanic populations, and it appears that its prevalence is lower in Hispanic populations compared to non-Hispanics despite the presence of a more adverse cardiovascular risk profile in the former (Figure 3-2 and Table 3-2).[26]

Table 3-2: Characteristics of Participants in MESA

	White (n=2,619)	Black (n=1,989)
Age (yr)	63.1 ± 10.3	63.0 ± 10.1
Women, %	51.9	55.5
BMI, kg/m^2	27.7 ± 5.1	30.2 ± 5.9
Systolic BP (mm Hg)	123.5 ± 20.4	131.7 ± 21.6
Diastolic BP (mm Hg)	70.2 ± 10.0	74.5 ± 10.2
Total cholesterol (mg/dL)	5.07 ± 0.91	4.91 ± 0.94
LDL cholesterol (mg/dL)	3.03 ± 0.78	3.01 ± 0.85
HDL cholesterol (mg/dL)	1.35 ± 0.41	1.36 ± 0.40
Triglycerides, mmol/L (mg/dL)	1.50 ± 1.02	1.19 ± 0.78
Smoking, %		
Current	11.6	18.0
Former	44.0	36.4
Never	44.4	45.6
Diabetes status, %		
Diabetic	7.8	20.6
Impaired fasting glucose	6.5	7.8
No diabetes	85.7	71.6
Hypertension, %	34.6	55.4
Use of antihypertensive medications, %	32.1	48.5

Comparison of conventional risk factors in MESA study (mean and SD are shown).

BP=blood pressure; BMI=body mass index; HDL=high-density lipoprotein; LDL=low-density lipoprotein. Data from references 21, 26.

Hispanic (n=1,494)	Chinese (n=803)
61.8 ± 10.4	62.9 ± 10.3
51.9	51.4
29.4 ± 5.1	24.0 ± 3.3
126.7 ± 21.9	124.6 ± 21.6
71.5 ± 10.1	72.0 ± 10.3
5.13 ± 0.97	4.99 ± 0.82
3.10 ± 0.85	2.98 ± 0.75
1.24 ± 0.34	1.28 ± 0.33
1.77 ± 1.14	1.61 ± 0.96
13.5	5.6
32.3	19.1
54.2	75.3
20.8	15.7
8.7	8.9
70.4	75.4
37.4	36.1
31.5	27.9

Based on these considerations, the traditional cardio-vascular risk factors pertaining to Hispanic populations are unlikely to differ fundamentally from those prevailing in the general US population. The idea of an authentic Hispanic paradox is not supported by evidence and much of it could be readily explained by acculturation and misclassification of individuals.

Risk Factors in American Indians

Epidemiologic Studies of Multiple Risk Factors

The Strong Heart Study (SHS) was designed to estimate cardiovascular disease (CVD) mortality and morbidity rates and the prevalence of known and suspected cardiovascular disease risk factors in American Indians.[27] The study population consisted of 12 tribes in three geographic areas: one area near Phoenix, Arizona, the southwestern area of Oklahoma, and the Aberdeen area of North and South Dakota. The study included three components: (a) a mortality survey to estimate CVD mortality rates for 1984 through 1988 among tribal members 35 to 74 years of age; (b) a morbidity survey to estimate incidence of both first and first or recurrent hospitalized MI and stroke (cerebrovascular disease) among tribal members 45-74 years of age in 1984-1988; and (c) a clinical examination of tribal members 45-74 years of age to estimate the prevalence of cardiovascular disease and its associations with risk factors. Family history, diet, alcohol and tobacco consumption, physical activity, degree of acculturation, and socioeconomic status were assessed. The physical examination included measurements of body fat, body circumferences, and blood pressure, cardiopulmonary examination, evaluation for PAD, and a 12-lead electro-cardiogram. Laboratory measurements included fasting and postload glucose, insulin, fasting lipids, apoproteins, fibrinogen, and glycosylated hemoglobin (HbA_{1c}). Also measured were serum and urine creatinine and urinary albumin. DNA from lymphocytes was isolated and stored for subsequent genetic studies.[27]

In terms of individual risk factors, the prevalence of smoking and hypertension was high compared to the general US population (Table 3-3). The prevalence of hypertension in Arizona and Oklahoma Indians was higher than that for the entire US.

In contrast to reports from non-Indian populations, diabetes was found to be the strongest risk factor[28] and its prevalence was highest in Arizona Indians at >60%. Overt diabetes, impaired glucose tolerance, and proteinuria were frequent; almost half of the Arizona Indians had micro- or macroalbuminuria, and 20% of Oklahoma and South and North Dakota Indians had significant proteinuria. Obesity was high in all three groups, with Arizona Indians having the highest rates and the highest mean body mass indices. The prevalence of alcohol use was lower among Indians than in the rest of the US, but binge drinking was common among those who used alcohol. Despite the presence of these risk factors the prevalence of MI was low compared to other populations.[29] It was also found that the distribution of the individual risk factors varied in certain respects between the groups of Indians studied.[29]

The subsequent surveillance of those enrolled in the study yielded interesting findings with respect to the incidence of CHD.[28] A total of 4,549 participants were followed for an average of 4.2 years (1991 to 1995), and 88% of those remaining alive underwent a second examination (1993 to 1995). The CVD morbidity and mortality rates were higher in men than in women and were similar in the three geographic areas. CHD incidence rates among American Indian men and women were *almost 2-fold* higher than those in the ARIC study. Significant independent predictors of CVD in women were diabetes, age, obesity (inverse), LDL cholesterol, albuminuria, triglycerides, and hypertension. In men, diabetes, age, LDL cholesterol,

Table 3-3: Age- and Center-Adjusted Hazard Rate Ratios for Fatal and Nonfatal CVD by Major CVD Risk Factors: Strong Heart Study[28]

Risk Factor	Women	Men
Hypertension	2.48	1.67
LDL Cholesterol	1.18	1.20
HDL Cholesterol	1.43	2.13
Diabetes mellitus	0.52	0.55
Current vs never smoker	1.58	1.08
Former vs never smoker	3.50	2.16
Insulin	1.13	1.24
Albuminuria		
Micro vs normal	2.38	1.65
Macro vs normal	5.36	3.81
Percentage body fat	0.46	0.64
Waist	0.94	0.97
Fibrinogen	2.38	1.84
Full-blooded Indian	1.06	0.94

HDL=high-density lipoprotein; LDL=low-density lipoprotein.

Mean of the lowest quartile group vs mean of the upper quartile group: 156 vs 74 mg/dL in women, 158 vs 74 mg/dL in men for LDL cholesterol; 66 vs 34 mg/dL in women, 61 vs 30 mg/dL in men for HDL cholesterol; 278 vs 66 mg/dL in women, 306 vs 61 mg/dL in men for triglycerides; 42.29 vs 7.31 µU/mL in women, 39.90 vs 5.24 µU/mL in men for insulin; 50% vs 32% in women, 37% vs 21% in men for percentage body fat; 127 cm vs 88 cm in women, 120 cm vs 88 cm in men for waist; and 416 vs 222 mg/dL in women, 387 vs 205 mg/dL in men for fibrinogen.

albuminuria, and hypertension were independent predictors of CVD.

The findings of the SHS taken collectively suggest that American Indians form a unique subgroup of the US population in which a significant proportion of the risk for CHD is derived from diabetes (with associated features such as microalbuminuria and proteinuria) and hypertension. When the Framingham/NCEP III algorithm was applied to American Indians, it overpredicted the number of events in women during a 5-year period.[30]

However, in a more recent study,[31] new prediction equations were developed for the SHS to predict CHD risk over a 10-year period. In this population with a high rate of diabetes and albuminuria, it was found that age, gender, total cholesterol, LDL cholesterol, HDL cholesterol, smoking, diabetes, hypertension, and albuminuria were significant CHD risk factors. A risk calculator is available on the Strong Heart Study web site, which provides predicted risk of CHD in 10 years with input of these risk factors[32] (http://strongheart.ouhsc.edu/CHDcalculator/calculator.html).

Peripheral Arterial Disease

In the SHS cohort, using the single criterion of an ankle brachial index <0.9, the prevalence of PAD was found to be approximately 5.3% across centers, with women having slightly higher rates than men. Multiple logistic regression analyses were used to predict PAD for women and men. Age, systolic blood pressure, current cigarette smoking, pack-years of smoking, albuminuria (micro- and macro-), LDL cholesterol level, and fibrinogen level were significantly positively associated with PAD. Current alcohol consumption was significantly negatively associated with PAD. In contrast to other groups, in American Indians, the association of albuminuria with PAD may equal or exceed the association of cigarette smoking with PAD. Not surprisingly, PAD was also associated with all-cause mortality in the population.[33]

Despite the fact that a significant number of studies have provided convincing evidence about the unique nature of the risk factors for CHD that operate in American Indians, there has been little progress in controlling them through preventive measures. The changes in the pattern of risk factors were examined in the SHS cohort over a 4-year period by Welty et al,[34] and they found that the incidence of diabetes and hypertension increased over this period while the changes observed in the other risk factors could best be described as modest, if any.

Risk Factors in Asian Populations

In the US, persons having origins in any of the original peoples of the Far East, Southeast Asia, or the Indian subcontinent are considered Asian. There are two main subgroups in this category: those designated as South Asian (from India, Pakistan, Bangladesh, and Sri Lanka) and ethnic Chinese and Japanese (from the Far East). There are several important differences in the interaction of conventional cardiovascular risk factors for CHD in these groups compared to Caucasian populations in the US.

South Asians

Epidemiology and Multiple Risk Factors

The findings in South Asian patients in the INTER-HEART study were analyzed in a substudy by Joshi et al.[35] They compared the cardiovascular risk factors in 1,732 South Asian patients who had suffered a first MI and 2,204 age- and gender-matched controls. The mean age of those who had sustained an MI was approximately 6 years lower in South Asian populations than in comparable groups in other countries. The prevalence of protective risk factors (leisure time physical activity, regular alcohol intake, and daily intake of fruits and vegetables) was markedly lower (all P <0.001) in both cases and controls in South Asian countries. Current and former smoking, history of hypertension, history of diabetes, high waist-to-hip ratio, elevated apolipoprotein B100 (ApoB$_{100}$)/apolipoprotein A-I (ApoA-I) ratio (top vs lowest tertile), and adverse psychosocial factors were strongly associated with increased risk of MI. Alcohol consumption was not found to be a risk factor in this population. Overall, the combined odds ratios for all nine risk factors were similar in native South Asians and in individuals from other countries. Thus, the population-attributable risk was 85.8% among native South Asians and 88.2% in individuals from other regions. After adjusting for the influence of other risk factors, the probability of experiencing MI at a young age was similar to that in other countries. Therefore, the earlier age of the first MI could be explained by the presence of higher risk factors at a young age (Figure 3-4).

Studies performed in the United Kingdom, US, Trinidad, and South Africa have confirmed a high rate of CVD among expatriate Indians, approaching 3-5 times that of native populations.[36,37] These differences exist despite the low overall prevalence of smoking, hypertension, and obesity in this group compared to other groups. This apparent discrepancy (the South Asian paradox) has been attributed to several factors that affect overall cardiovascular risk: (a) although the conventional lipid parameters are acceptable, concentrations of Lp(a) have been consistently elevated compared to those of Caucasians[38]; (b) low percentage of large HDL particles despite normal concentrations of HDL cholesterol[39]; and (c) greater sensitivity to saturated dietary fat (lipid profiles in the normal range despite a lower-than-normal consumption of dietary fat).[40]

Carotid Ultrasound and Coronary Artery Calcification

Because of the perception that there is a higher incidence of CHD in South Asians living in the US, there has been an increasing interest to diagnose subclinical disease in this group by detecting carotid atherosclerosis or coronary calcification. These studies have yielded information that provides support for an altered interaction

71

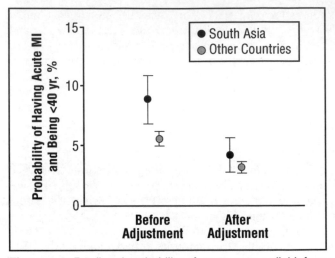

Figure 3-4: Predicted probability of acute myocardial infarction (MI) at a younger age in South Asians compared with individuals from other countries. This analysis was performed among acute MI cases only. Before adjustment for the nine risk factors, there was a higher probability of cases in patients who were younger than 40 years in the South Asian group compared with cases from other countries (*P*=0.001). However, after adjustment for these risk factors, the difference in probabilities of predicted cases of acute MI in younger persons was attenuated and not statistically significant (*P*=0.27). Error bars indicate 95% confidence intervals.[35]

of conventional cardiovascular risk factors in this population. Chow et al[41] compared the effects of risk factors on carotid intima-media thickness (IMT) in a population of South Asians in randomly selected adults from two villages in rural India (n=303) compared to sampled adults from Australia (n=1,111). There were stronger associations of cholesterol (*P* for interaction=0.009) and diabetes (*P*=0.04) with carotid IMT in the Indian compared to the Australian population. Also, while increasing HDL cholesterol was associated with decreasing carotid IMT in the

Australian population, the reverse was true for the Indian population (*P* <0.001). The associations of IMT with blood pressure, triglycerides, age, HDL-to-total cholesterol ratio, glucose, body mass index (BMI), waist, waist-to-hip ratio, and smoking were not different between the populations. Greater adverse effects of total cholesterol and diabetes on atherosclerosis and the absence of a protective effect of HDL cholesterol among Asian Indians provide a possible novel explanation for observed excess rates of CVD in this group.

However, in a cross-sectional population study of 1,015 Canadian adults of caucasian European, South Asian, Chinese, and aboriginal ancestry, CHD risk was calculated by the 10-year FRS and 752 (74%) participants were classified as low risk.[42] Of these, 175 (23%) had evidence of subclinical atherosclerosis (carotid IMT ≥75th percentile adjusted for age, sex, and ethnicity). Independent predictors of carotid atherosclerosis in low-risk subjects included female sex, systolic blood pressure, and high apolipoprotein B. The proportion of individuals with subclinical atherosclerosis in the low-risk groups was similar in all ethnic groups examined.

The second area of subclinical atherosclerosis that has been investigated is calcification of the coronary arteries. Hawalkar et al[43] compared the prevalence of coronary artery calcification in a group of age-matched Caucasians and minorities living in the US (Table 3-4). All patients were asymptomatic and were referred for evaluation of coronary artery calcification. All the minority groups had a greater prevalence of diabetes and had a less frequent family history of CHD than did the Caucasians. The Asian Indians did not have a higher prevalence of diabetes, metabolic syndrome, and hyperlipidemia. They were younger and their blood pressures were lower, but they had the highest degree of coronary calcification (97% in those >60 years). Thus, it was concluded that South Asians have a higher prevalence of CHD that manifests itself at a

Table 3-4: Prevalence (%) of Risk Factors in Asian Indians Living in the US Compared to Other Ethnic Groups[43]

	Caucasian	Asian Indian	Hispanic	African American	Asian
Age (years)	56	52	53	56	56
Men	58	59	56	60	60
Hypertension	28	22	33	51	36
Tobacco	8	8	8	12	9
Diabetes mellitus	6	18	13	15	15
Hypercho-lesterolemia	39	35	35	33	40
Family history	64	48	50	47	43

younger age than in Caucasians. HDL cholesterol does not appear to have the same protective effect as it does in Caucasians living in the US. Also, Lp(a) may be a significant risk factor in this population. There is probably sufficient data available to conclude that subclinical atherosclerosis should be routinely sought in this group if the Lp(a) concentration is high and if the HDL fractionation shows a reduced concentration of large particles.

Chinese

The largest epidemiologic study of cardiovascular risk factors in Chinese is the Chinese Multi-province Cohort Study (CMCS).[44] A total of 30,121 Chinese participants 35 to 64 years of age were included in the original CMCS cohort and 3,118 participants from Beijing were added in

1996 and 1999. In all, 16,552 participants were followed until the end of 2002. Liu et al compared the Framingham algorithm for predicting CHD in this population together with a new algorithm derived solely from the Chinese data set. The overall methodology used was similar to that employed in the Framingham Study. Although the risk factors themselves were similar, their interactions were found to be somewhat different. The ability to discriminate between people who develop CHD and those who do not in the CMCS cohort was similar whether one used the Framingham functions or the unique functions derived from the CMCS cohort. The area under the receiver operating characteristic curve was 0.705 for men and 0.742 for women, using the Framingham functions, compared to 0.736 for men and 0.759 for women using the CMCS functions. However, the original Framingham functions systematically overestimated the absolute CHD risk in the CMCS cohort. Recalibration of the Framingham functions using the mean values of risk factors and mean CHD incidence rates of the CMCS cohort substantially improved the performance of the Framingham functions in the CMCS cohort. However, when the algorithm obtained from the CMCS cohort was applied directly, there was a greater degree of concordance between the predicted incidence and the actual incidence of CHD events (Figure 3-5).

Lipids, Hypertension, Obesity, Smoking, and PAD

Only a few large studies have addressed the prevalence of cardiovascular risk factors in Chinese living in the US. The Multi-Ethnic Study of Atherosclerosis (MESA)[43-45] reported that the prevalence of obesity and smoking was least in Asians (Chinese). Other factors, such as serum lipids[45] and hypertension,[46] were similar to those recorded in Caucasians. The prevalence of PAD[47] and subclinical atherosclerosis in the form of coronary calcification[48] were also lower in Chinese compared to Caucasians.

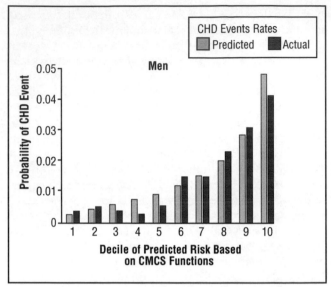

Figure 3-5: Ten-year prediction of CHD events in CMCS men and women using the CMCS functions. CMCS indicates Chinese Multi-provincial Cohort Study. Coronary heart disease (CHD) events included coronary death and myocardial infarction.[44]

Japanese

Comparative Risk Factors in Japan and the US

Of all the Asian groups living in the US, the Japanese population is perhaps the group that has the longest experience of acculturation. In Japan, CHD incidence and mortality appear to be substantially lower at all ages than in the US despite an increase in serum total cholesterol, high smoking rate, and frequency of adverse blood pressure levels. The INTERLIPID study compared risk factors for CHD and dietary variables in Japanese living in Japan and 3rd- and 4th-generation Japanese emigrants living a primarily Western lifestyle in Hawaii.[49] Men and women 40 to 59 years of age were examined by common standardized methods—four samples in Japan (574 men, 571 women) and a Japanese-American sample in Hawaii (136 men, 131 women). Average systolic and diastolic blood pressures were significantly higher in men in Japan than in Hawaii; there were no significant differences in women. The treatment rate of hypertension was much lower in Japan than Hawaii. Smoking prevalence was higher, markedly so for men, in Japan than Hawaii. Body mass index, serum total and LDL cholesterol, HbA_{1c}, and fibrinogen were significantly lower and HDL cholesterol was higher in Japan than in Hawaii. Total and saturated fat intakes were lower and polyunsaturated fatty acid and ω-3 fatty acid intakes were higher in Japan than in Hawaii. These differences, which were smaller for women than men, could partly explain the lower incidence of CHD and mortality in Japan than in the US.

The Honolulu Heart Study, one of the largest to address cardiovascular risk factors in Japanese Americans, was a prospective investigation of the association between a variety of baseline lifestyle and biologic factors in a middle-aged cohort of Japanese-American men (N = 2,710 between 55 and 64 years of age) and the 20-year incidence rates of total atherosclerotic end points, including fatal and nonfatal CHD, angina pectoris, thromboembolic strokes, and aortic aneurysms. After adjustment for each of the baseline characteristics examined, significant positive associations between quartile cutoffs of BMI, systolic blood pressure, serum levels of cholesterol, triglycerides, glucose, and uric acid, as well as cigarette smoking, and the occurrence of any atherosclerotic end point were seen. An inverse association was observed with alcohol consumption.[50] Not surprisingly, abnormal serum lipids were significant risk factors for developing CHD in noninsulin dependent diabetes.[51] It was also observed that the conventional cardiovascular risk factors observed at baseline were predictive of developing an abnormal brachial artery index 20 years later.[52]

Table 3-5: Distribution, Range, and Percentiles of CAC Scores for 311 Japanese Men in Japan and 300 Japanese Men in Hawaii Aged 40–50 Years From 2001 to 2005[53]

CAC	Japan		Hawaii	
	N	%	N	%
0	214	68.8	152	50.7
>0	97	31.2	148	49.3
10	36	11.6	96	32.0
100	7	2.3	40	13.3
≥400	2	0.6	10	3.3
1,000	0	0.0	3	1.0

CAC=coronary artery calcification (Agatson Score).

Despite the similarity of the risk factors in Japanese Americans and the general US population, the differences in the incidence of CHD mentioned in this chapter are also reflected in markers of subclinical coronary atherosclerosis. A cross-sectional study comparing Japanese men living in Japan and Japanese men living in Hawaii found that despite a worse risk factor profile in the former, the prevalence of coronary artery calcification was lower (Table 3-5).[53] As observed previously, the diets were significantly higher in saturated fats and lower in ω-3 unsaturated fatty acids in Japanese Americans.

Summary

Overall, the risk factors for CHD established by the Framingham Study apply to all special groups in the US, although there are differences in the precise interactions between individual factors within each major ethnic group. In African Americans, hypertension is a particularly important issue, while in American Indians diabetes with renal damage appears to play a significant role. South Asians appear to develop conventional cardiovascular risk factors at an earlier age than do other ethnic groups. The Chinese, Japanese, and Hispanics living in the US seem to have similar risk factor profiles to the general US population, but the incidence of CHD appears to be lowest in the former while the latter groups show the greatest effect of acculturation during their integration with the general US population.

References

1.   Abbott RD: The probability of developing certain cardiovascular diseases in eight years at specified values of some characteristics: The Framingham Study. In Kannel WB, Wolf PA, Garrison RJ, eds: The Framingham Study: An epidemiological investigation of cardiovascular disease. *National Technical Information Service. Springfield VA No BP 87-221644/A5.* 1987, Section 37.

2.   Wilson PW, D'Agostino RB, Levy D, et al: Prediction of coronary heart disease using risk factor categories. *Circulation* 1998;97:1837-1847.

3.   The fifth report of the Joint National Committee on Detection, Evaluation, and Treatment of High Blood Pressure (JNC V): *Arch Intern Med* 1993;153:154-183.

4.   Expert Panel on Detection and Treatment of High Blood Cholesterol in Adults. Executive summary of the Third Report of the National Cholesterol Education Program (NCEP) Expert Panel on Detection, Evaluation and Treatment of High Blood Cholesterol in Adults (Adult Treatment Panel III). *JAMA* 2001;285:2486-2497.

5.   Grundy SM, Cleeman JL, Merz CN, et al: Implications of recent clinical trials for the National Cholesterol Education Program Adult Treatment Panel III Guidelines. *J Am Coll Cardiol* 2004;44: 720-732.

6.   Jackson R: Updated New Zealand cardiovascular risk-benefit prediction guide. *BMJ* 2000;320:709-710.

7.   Conroy RM, Pyorala K, Fitzgerald AP, et al: Estimation of ten-year risk of fatal cardiovascular diease in Europe: The SCORE project. *Eur Heart J* 2003;24:987-1003.

8.   Zhang XF, Attia J, D'Este C, et al: A risk score predicted coronary heart disease and stroke in a Chinese cohort. *J Clin Epidemiol* 2005;58:951-958.

9.   Hippsley-Cox J, Coupland C, Vinogradova Y, et al: Derivation and validation of QRISK, a new cardiovascular disease risk score for the United Kingdom: prospective open cohort study. *BMJ* 2007:335:136.

10.   Woodward Brindle P, Tinstall-Pedoe H: Adding social deprivation and family history to cardiovascular risk assessment: the ASSIGN score from the Scottish Heart Health Extended Cohort (SHHEC). *Heart* 2007;93:172-176.

11.   Yusuf S, Hawken S, Ounpuu S, et al: Effect of potentially modifiable risk factors associated with myocardial infarction in 52 countries (the INTERHEART study): case-control study. *Lancet* 2004;364:937-952.

12.   Crook ED, Clark BL, Bradford ST, et al: From 1960s Evans County Georgia to present-day Jackson, Mississippi: an exploration of the evolution of cardiovascular disease in African Americans. *Am J Med Sci* 2003;325:307-314.

13.   The Atherosclerosis Risk in Communities (ARIC) Study: design and objectives. *Am J Epidemiol* 1989;129:687-702.

14.   Taylor HA Jr, Wilson JG, Jones DW, et al: Toward resolution of cardiovascular health disparities in African Americans: design and methods of the Jackson Heart Study. *Ethn Dis* 2005;15(4 suppl 6): S6-S17.

15.   Chambless LE, Folsom AR, Sharrett AR, et al: Coronary heart disease risk prediction in the Atherosclerosis Risk in Communities (ARIC) study. *J Clin Epidemiol* 2003;56:880-890.

16.   O'Meara KS, Kardia SL, Armon JJ, et al: Ethnic and sex differences in the prevalence, treatment, and control of dyslipidemia among hypertensive adults in the GENOA Study. *Arch Intern Med* 2004;164:1313-1318.

17.   Kullo IJ, Jan MF, Bailey KR, et al: Ethnic differences in low-density lipoprotein particle size in hypertensive adults. *J Clin Lipidol* 2007;1:218-224.

18. Benton JL Blumenthal RS, Becker DM, et al: Predictors of low-density lipoprotein particle size in a high-risk African-American population. *Am J Cardiol* 2005;95:1320-1323.

19. Hallman DM, Brown SA, Ballantyne CM, et al: Relationship between low-density lipoprotein subclasses and asymptomatic atherosclerosis in subjects from the Atherosclerosis Risk in Communities (ARIC) Study. *Biomarkers* 2004;9:190-202.

20. Teo KK, Onupuu S, Hawken S, et al, and the INTERHEART Study Investigators: Tobacco use and risk of myocardial infarction in 52 countries in the INTERHEART study: a case-control study. *Lancet* 2006;368:647-658.

21. Centers for Disease Control and Prevention: Adult cigarette smoking in the United States: current estimates. Accessed at: http://www.cdc.gov/tobacco/data_statistics/fact_sheets/adult_data/cig_smoking/index.htm.

22. Nelson KM, Reiber G, Kohler T, et al: Peripheral arterial disease in a multiethnic national sample: the role of conventional risk factors and allostatic load. *Ethn Dis* 2007;17:669-675.

23. Ix JH, Allison MA, Denenberg JO, et al: Novel cardiovascular risk factors do not completely explain the higher prevalence of peripheral arterial disease among African Americans. The San Diego Population Study. *J Am Coll Cardiol* 2008;51:2347-2354.

24. Smith DP, Bradshaw BS: Rethinking the Hispanic paradox: Death rates and life expectancy for US non-Hispanic white and Hispanic populations. *Am J Public Health* 2006;96:1686-1692.

25. Lerman-Garber I, Villa AR, Caballero E: Diabetes and cardiovascular disease. Is there a true Hispanic paradox? *Rev Invest Clin* 2004;56:282-296.

26. Bild DE, Detrano R, Peterson D, et al: Ethnic differences in coronary calcification: the Multi-Ethnic Study of Atherosclerosis (MESA). *Circulation* 2005;111:1313-1320.

27. Lee ET, Welty TK, Fabsitz R, et al: The Strong Heart Study. A study of cardiovascular disease in American Indians: design and methods. *Am J Epidemiol* 1990;132:1141-1155.

28. Howard BV, Lee ET, Cowan LD, et al: Rising tide of cardiovascular disease in American Indians. The Strong Heart Study. *Circulation* 1999;99:2389-2395.

29.   Welty TK, Lee ET, Yeh J, et al: Cardiovascular disease risk factors among American Indians. The Strong Heart Study. *Am J Epidemiol* 1995;142:269-287.

30.   D'Agostino RB Sr, Grundy S, Sullivan LM, Wilson P; CHD Risk Prediction Group: Validation of the Framingham coronary heart disease prediction scores: results of a multiple ethnic groups investigation. *JAMA* 2001;286:180-187.

31.   Lee ET, Howard BV, Wang W, et al: Prediction of coronary heart disease in a population with high prevalence of diabetes and albuminuria: the Strong Heart Study. *Circulation* 2006;113:2897-2905.

32.   Strong Heart Study: Calculator: estimated risk of developing CHD in 10 years, 2006. Accessed at: http://strongheart.ouhsc.edu/CHDcalculator/calculator.html.

33.   Resnick HE, Lindsay RS, McDermott MM, et al: Relationship of high and low ankle brachial index to all-cause and cardiovascular disease mortality: the Strong Heart Study. *Circulation* 2004;109:733-739.

34.   Welty TK, Rhoades DA, Yeh F, et al: Changes in cardiovascular disease risk factors among American Indians. The Strong Heart Study. *Ann Epidemiol* 2002;12:97-106.

35.   Joshi P, Islam S, Pais P, et al: Risk factors for early myocardial infarction in South Asians compared with individuals in other countries. *JAMA* 2007;297:286-294.

36.   Vardan S, Mookherjee S, Vardan S, et al: Special features of coronary heart disease of the peoples of the Indian sub-continent. *Indian Heart J* 1995;47:399-407.

37.   Venkata C, Ram S: Hypertension and other cardiac risk factors among Asian Indians. *Am J Hypertens* 1995;8:124S-127S.

38.   Anand SS, Enas EA, Pogue J, et al: Elevated lipoprotein(a) levels in South Asians in North America. *Metabolism* 1998;47:182-184.

39.   Bhalodkar NC, Blum S, Rana T, et al: Comparison of levels of large and small high-density lipoprotein cholesterol in Asian Indian men compared with Caucasian men in the Framingham Offspring Study. *Am J Cardiol* 2004;94:1561-1563.

40.   Singh RB, Niaz MA, Ghosh S, et al: Low fat intake and coronary artery disease in a population with higher prevalence of coronary artery disease: The Indian paradox. *J Am Coll Nutr* 1998;17:342-350.

41.   Chow CK, McQuillan B, Raju PK, et al: Greater adverse effects of cholesterol and diabetes on carotid intima-media thickness in South Asian Indians: comparison of risk factor-IMT associations in two population-based surveys. *Atherosclerosis* 2008;199:116-122.

42.   Grewal J, Anand S, Islam S, Lonn E; SHARE and SHARE-AP Investigators: Prevalence and predictors of subclinical atherosclerosis among asymptomatic "low risk" individuals in a multiethnic population. *Atherosclerosis* 2008;197:435-442.

43.   Hawalkar NA, Agrawal N, Reiss DS, et al: Comparison of prevalence and severity of coronary calcium determined by electron beam tomography in various ethnic groups. *Am J Cardiol* 2003; 91:1225.

44.   Liu J, Hong Y, D'Agostino RB, et al: Predictive value for the Chinese population of the Framingham CHD Risk Assessment Tool compared with the Chinese Multi-provincial Cohort Study. *JAMA* 2004;291:2591-2599.

45.   Goff DC Jr, Bertoni AG, Kramer H, et al: Dyslipidemia prevalence, treatment, and control in the Multi-Ethnic Study of Atherosclerosis (MESA): gender, ethnicity, and coronary artery calcium. *Circulation* 2006;113:647-656.

46.   Kramer H, Han C, Post W, et al: Racial/ethnic differences in hypertension and hypertension treatment and control in the multi-ethnic study of atherosclerosis (MESA). *Am J Hypertens* 2004;17: 963-970.

47.   Allison MA, Criqui MH, McClelland RL, et al: The effect of novel cardiovascular risk factors on the ethnic-specific odds for peripheral arterial disease in the Multi-Ethnic Study of Atherosclerosis (MESA). *J Am Coll Cardiol* 2006;48:1190-1197.

48.   Budoff MJ, Nasir K, Mao S, et al: Ethnic differences of the presence and severity of coronary atherosclerosis. *Atherosclerosis* 2006;187:343-350.

49.   Ueshima H, Saitoh S, Nakagawa H, et al, for the INTERLIPID Research Group: Differences in cardiovascular disease risk factors between Japanese in Japan and Japanese-Americans in Hawaii: the INTERLIPID study. *J Hum Hypertens* 2003;17:631-639.

50.   Goldberg RJ, Benfante R, Chiu D, et al: Lifestyle and biologic factors associated with atherosclerotic disease in middle-aged men. 20-year findings from the Honolulu Heart Program. *Arterioscler Thromb Vasc Biol* 1996;16:1495-1500.

51. Laws A, Marcus EB, Grove JS, et al: Lipids and lipoproteins as risk factors for coronary heart disease in men with abnormal glucose tolerance: the Honolulu Heart Program. *J Intern Med* 1993;234: 471-478.

52. Curb JD, Masaki K, Rodriguez BL, et al: Peripheral artery disease and cardiovascular risk factors in the elderly. The Honolulu Heart Program. *Arterioscler Thromb Vasc Biol* 1996;16:1495-1500.

53. Abbott RD, Ueshima H, Rodriguez BL, et al: Coronary artery calcification in Japanese men in Japan and Hawaii. *Am J Epidemiol* 2007;166:1280-1287.

Chapter 4

Hypertension

By Philip R. Liebson, MD

Racial differences in blood pressure were reported as early as 1932 when investigators found that systolic blood pressure recorded in 6,000 black workmen was 7 mm Hg higher than in 8,000 white workmen in New Orleans.[1] Even though hypertension is an important contributor to cardiovascular disease (CVD), recent surveys indicate that less than one-third of the hypertensive population in the United States has adequate blood pressure control, despite the availability of a large variety of antihypertensive medications.[2] In fact, hypertension prevalence is increasing, by 3.7% from 1988-1991 to 1999-2000 based on National Health and Nutrition Examination Survey (NHANES) surveys.[2] Although almost 70% of persons were aware of their hypertension in the more recent survey, and almost 60% were being treated (an increase of 6% from the earlier survey), hypertension was controlled in only 31% (an increase of slightly over 6%). In terms of special populations, women, the elderly (more than 60 years of age) and Mexican Americans had lower rates of control than men, younger persons, and non-Hispanic whites (Table 4-1).

A more recent sampling comparing expanded sample sizes of NHANES (1998-1994 vs 1999-2002) provided further information regarding race-specific data on hypertension comparing blacks with whites.[3] The prevalence of hypertension was highest in blacks, increasing from 36%

Table 4-1: Awareness, Treatment, and Control of Hypertension by Age in the US Population 1988-2000[a]

Age yr	Prevalence, % (SE) 1988-1991	Prevalence, % (SE) 1991-1994
18-39	61.5(4.5)	49.1 (6.9)[b]
40-59	73.2 (2.4)	72.7 (3.3)
≥60	68.3(1.3)	69.1 (1.6)
18-39	34.1 (5.4)	24.8 (3.5)[b]
40-59	53.9 (2.7)	54.2 (2.4)
≥60	55.1 (1.2)	56.7 (1.6)
18-39	61.5 (7.2)[b]	70.2 (7.4)[b]
40-59	53.7 (3.4)[c]	54.2 (3.6)[c]
≥60	40.8 (2.8)	35.2 (2.2)
18-39	21.0 (5.2)	17.4 (3.1)[b]
40-59	28.9 (2.4)	29.4 (2.4)[c]
≥60	22.5 (1.7)	20.0 (1.6)

[a]Data are weighted to the US population.

[b]Estimates are unreliable because of National Health and Nutrition Examination Survey minimum sample size criteria or coefficient of variation of at least 0.30.

[c]$P <0.01$ for the difference among groups within the same survey (age ≥60 years as the referent).

1999-2000	Change 1988-2000 % (95% CI)	P Value
Awareness		
51.8 (5.8)[b]	-9.7 (-24.1–4.7)	NA
73.3 (2.8)	0.1 (-7.1 –7.3)	.49
69.8 (1.9)	1.5 (-3.0–6.0)	.26
Treatment		
27.7 (5.3)[b]	-6.4 (-21.2– 8.4)	NA
62.9 (3.1)	9.0 (0.9 –17.1)	.01
62.7 (2.0)	7.6 (-4.5 –10.3)	.006
Control (all treated)		
51.9 (11.5)[b]	-9.6 (-36.2 – 17.0)	NA
66.4 (3.7)[d]	12.7 (2.9–22.5)	.006
43.7 (2.5)	2.9 (-4.5 –10.3)	.22
Control (all hypertensive)		
14.4 (4.3)[b]	-6.6 (-19.8 – 6.6)	NA
41.6 (3.2)[d]	12.7 (4.9 – 20.5)	<.001
27.4 (1.8)	4.9 (0–9.8)	.02

[d] $P < 0.001$ for the difference among groups within the same survey (age ≥60 years as the referent)

CI=confidence interval, NA=not applicable due to unreliable data, SE=standard error.

From Hajjar[2] with permission.

to 41% in the earlier NHANES survey to the later one (and from 24%-29% among whites).[3] However, awareness of their hypertension status was higher in blacks (78% vs 70%), an increase of 4% for blacks since the earlier survey, without a change of awareness among whites. Treatment increased in blacks from 58% to 68%. Although blood pressure control in blacks increased from 23% to 32% since the earlier survey, it remained below whites in both surveys, with 35% of whites being under blood pressure control in the latter survey.

In the 1999-2004 NHANES survey, the prevalence of hypertension increased with age, from 7.3% in those 18-39 years of age, to 66.3% in those ≥60 years.[4] The blood pressure control rate (to <140/90 mm Hg) increased from 29.2% in 1999-2000 to 36.8% in 2003-2004. This increase was significant in both sexes, blacks, and Mexican Americans.

In the Multi-Ethnic Study of Atherosclerosis (MESA) involving 6,814 adults without clinical heart disease, the prevalence of hypertension or self-reported treatment of hypertension was significantly higher in blacks than in whites (60% vs 38%)[5] (Figure 4-1). After adjustment for age, body mass index (BMI), presence of diabetes and smoking, blacks as well as those of Chinese ethnicity were associated with higher prevalence of hypertension compared with whites, and socioeconomic factors were significantly associated with treated but uncontrolled hypertension in blacks compared with other racial groups.

In a study of adherence to guidelines, in this case the Sixth Report of the Joint National Committee on Prevention, Detection, Evaluation, and Treatment of High Blood Pressure (JNC 6) guidelines of 1997, a review of medical records of 15,768 visits to 12 internal medicine clinics in 2001-2002 revealed greater physician adherence among blacks (84%) and Hispanics (83%) than whites (78%) (P <0.001).[6] On the other hand, blood pressure was controlled most among whites (39%) compared to 35% for blacks and 33% for Hispanics (P <0.001). However, in all

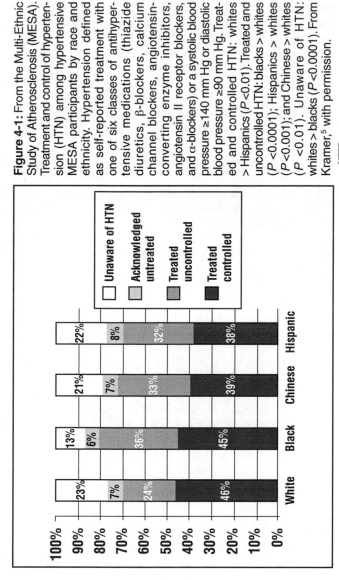

Figure 4-1: From the Multi-Ethnic Study of Atherosclerosis (MESA). Treatment and control of hypertension (HTN) among hypertensive MESA participants by race and ethnicity. Hypertension defined as self-reported treatment with one of six classes of antihypertensive medications (thiazide diuretics, β-blockers, calcium channel blockers, angiotensin-converting enzyme inhibitors, angiotensin II receptor blockers, and α-blockers) or a systolic blood pressure ≥140 mm Hg or diastolic blood pressure ≥90 mm Hg. Treated and controlled HTN: whites > Hispanics (P <0.01). Treated and uncontrolled HTN: blacks > whites (P <0.0001); Hispanics > whites (P <0.001); and Chinese > whites (P <0.01). Unaware of HTN: whites > blacks (P <0.0001). From Kramer,[5] with permission.

4

groups, intensification of therapy led to better control of blood pressure, although Hispanics were less likely than blacks and non-Hispanic whites to have blood pressure therapy intensified.

There appears to be a lack of substantial geographical difference in hypertension awareness comparing the 'stroke belt' region (southeastern US) with the country as a whole in racial assessment.[7] However, there appears to be a trend toward better treatment and control in the stroke belt region.

The prevalence of hypertension is as high as 65% in persons more than 60 years of age. Increasing BMI, an epidemic in this country, was independently associated with increased rates of hypertension. However, further analysis of the two NHANES surveys indicated that only 2.0% to 3.6% of the increase in hypertension prevalence was due to increase in BMI.[3,4] The increase in the diagnosis of hypertension may have also been due to the lower blood pressure indication for antihypertensive therapy in diabetics (130/85 vs 140/90) and, indeed, exclusion of diabetics from the analysis demonstrated that the increase in prevalence was not statistically significant. The latter NHANES survey indicated that almost 75% of all diabetics with hypertension did not have blood pressure controlled to <130/85 mm Hg.[8] This underscores the health problem of uncontrolled hypertension in the US, particularly in patients with diabetes, especially since blacks have a higher prevalence of diabetes than whites.

Differential access to health care may contribute to racial differences in blood pressure control. The Veterans Affairs (VA) system provides access to health care across racial and economic boundaries. A study of blood pressure control (<140/90 mm Hg) in a VA versus non-VA setting in the Southeastern US (mostly South Carolina) found that blood pressure control was higher in blacks in a VA setting compared to a non-VA setting (49.4% vs 44.0%) after controlling for age, comorbid conditions, and rural-urban classification.[9] No differences were seen among white men in both settings, but even in a VA setting white men had a higher control rate (55.6%) than black men, even though blacks had similar numbers of prescriptions and more visits at VA sites than did whites. Although antihypertensive treatments are examined fully later in this chapter, it would be worthwhile to review the antihypertensive medications prescribed in the VA versus non-VA study, which covered the period between 2001 and 2003. In both settings, a higher percentage of blacks received diuretics and dihydropyridine calcium channel blockers (CCBs), which is to be expected based on the evidence of greater success in lowering blood pressure in blacks with these classes of agents. However, a similar percentage of blacks and whites received angiotensin-converting enzyme (ACE) inhibitors in the VA setting, and of further interest, ACE inhibitors were prescribed in a higher percentage of blacks than whites in the non-VA setting. The better blood pressure control rate of blacks in the VA versus non-VA setting could only be explained by the greater number of visits of blacks to VA versus non-VA sites, possibly because of insurance issues, prescription costs, and other socioeconomic barriers at non-VA sites.

The importance of physician counseling was evaluated in another VA study of 460 black and 333 white hypertensive patients from three urban tertiary VA medical centers.[10] Although the results showed no racial disparity in blood pressure control, blacks received more counseling, and the association of physician behavior with blood pressure control was not mediated by trust in the physician, although whites showed more trust in the physician than did blacks.

Hypertension is not predominantly a condition of the elderly. Based on NHANES 1999-2002, 63% of black adults and 45% of white adults with hypertension are under 60 years of age.[3] However, treatment rates are significantly higher in blacks than in whites (68% vs 60%), mostly based on the higher treatment rates of black women compared to white women. Nonetheless, blood pressure control remains lower in blacks than in whites.

Although the NHANES surveys provide important cross-sectional assessments of the awareness, prevalence, and treatment response of hypertension in the general population, they omit persons in nursing homes and other institutions, include only Mexican Americans among the Hispanic population, and restrict analysis to participants who have blood pressure measurements taken during a specific visit and not hypertensives who do not have a blood pressure taken during the visit.[11] In addition, participants who have been told they have hypertension but have blood pressures below 140/90 and were not receiving medications were not counted as hypertensive.[2] Presumably, a higher prevalence would be found if these factors were taken into account.

Differences in prevalence rates among various groups may depend on genetic and socioeconomic factors. Hispanics, for example, are less likely to have a regular health-care physician and insurance than either blacks or whites,[12] and hypertensive blacks are less likely to have health insurance compared to whites.[3] Although this was found to be a significant factor in blood pressure control in persons under Medicare age (evaluation of persons 20-59), it still did not completely explain the significant racial disparity of blood pressure control in younger blacks versus whites.[3]

Ethnic Differences in Blood Pressure Management

Physician and patient attitudes can affect the degree of control of hypertension in individual patients. Although there may be some differences in interracial responses to some classes of antihypertensive agents, the aggressiveness of treatment intervention and willingness of the patient to adhere to therapeutic recommendations must also be considered. Valuable information on interracial responses to antihypertensive interventions has been obtained from assessment of clinical trial results. This section will evaluate specific hypertension clinical trial results in relation to racial groups.

Blacks

Black hypertensives have been found to respond better to CCBs and diuretics than to ACE inhibitors and β-blockers.[13,14] More specific information from pertinent clinical trials involving black hypertensives is reviewed below.

ALLHAT

In the Antihypertensive and Lipid-Lowering Treatment to Prevent Heart Attack Trial (ALLHAT), which included chlorthalidone, lisinopril, amlodipine, and doxazosin, 15,094 blacks were included (35% of patients).[15] The primary outcome measure was combined nonfatal myocardial infarction (MI) and fatal coronary heart disease (CHD). No separate data were obtained for black patients in the doxazosin arm, halted after an interim analysis demonstrated increased adverse outcomes. However, blacks achieved a greater magnitude of benefit from thiazide diuretics in reduction of stroke, end-stage renal disease (ESRD), heart failure, and cardiovascular events than did nonblacks, without differences in CHD outcomes.[16] This was associated with a *4/1 mm Hg greater* blood pressure reduction in the chlorthalidone group versus the lisinopril group even when results were adjusted for blood pressure differences between groups.

LIFE

The Losartan Intervention for Endpoint Reduction in Hypertension (LIFE) study, which tested losartan versus atenolol, evaluated the effect of an angiotensin-receptor blocker (ARB) and β-blocker on composite end points of cardiovascular death, nonfatal stroke, and nonfatal MI.[17,18] All patients had ECG evidence of left ventricular hypertrophy (LVH) as an inclusion criterion. Only 6% of patients (533) were black. Blacks receiving losartan had a trend toward greater risk (RR 1.55, CI 1.00-1.28) compared with atenolol, in comparison with reduced risk in whites despite a greater regression of LVH[18] (Figure 4-2). Although the primary composite end point, incidence rates, in blacks was similar in each treatment group, thereafter the crude incidence rates in those receiving atenolol appeared to decline, with 4-year incidence of 9.7% for those on atenolol and 15.3% with those on losartan. However, blood pressure reduction was similar in blacks and whites. The conclusion drawn was that black patients might not respond as favorably to ARBs compared to nonblacks, with respect to cardiovascular outcomes.

AASK

The African American Study of Kidney Disease and Hypertension (AASK) compared the effects of an ACE inhibitor (ramipril), CCB (amlodipine), and β-blocker (metoprolol) on 1,094 hypertensive black patients with decreased glomerular filtration rates (GFR).[19,20] Patients were randomly assigned to one of these three agents and to one of two mean arterial pressure goals, 102–107 mm Hg ("usual" target goal) or ≤92 mm Hg ("lower" target goal). The primary outcome was the composite of rate of change of GFR, development of ESRD, and death.

Blood pressure achieved in the "usual" target group averaged 141/85 mm Hg and 128/78 mm Hg in the "lower" target group. The mean slope of decrease in GFR over 4 years did not change significantly between the "usual" and "lower" blood pressure group.[19] The lower blood pressure goal did not significantly affect the primary composite clinical outcome. The ACE inhibitor group, however, demonstrated a risk reduction in the primary outcome compared with the β-blocker (RR 0.78, P=0.04) and the CCB (RR 0.62, P=0.004), with no difference between the β-blocker and CCB. None of the drug group comparisons showed a significant effect on GFR slope. Proteinuria was slightly but not significantly lower in the "lower" blood pressure group

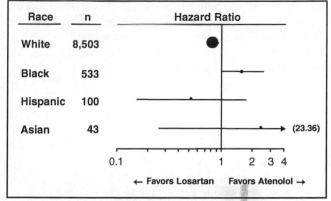

Race	n	Hazard Ratio
White	8,503	
Black	533	
Hispanic	100	
Asian	43	(23.36)

0.1   1   2   3   4

← Favors Losartan   Favors Atenolol →

Figure 4-2: From the Losartan Intervention for Endpoint Reduction in Hypertension (LIFE) study. Results of primary composite end point by ethnic group. The *dots* represent the hazard ratio; the *dot size* is proportional to the number of patients in each ethnic group, as shown to the *left.* The *line through each dot* corresponds to the 95% confidence interval. From Julius,[18] with permission.

compared with the "usual" blood pressure group (*P*=0.06). Over the 4-year period, proteinuria increase was greater in the CCB group than in the β-blocker and ramipril groups. In the secondary combined outcomes of renal failure and death, the ACE inhibitor significantly reduced this outcome compared with the CCB.[20] The results of this complex study demonstrated no additional slowing of the progression of hypertensive nephrosclerosis in the "lower" blood pressure group.[19] In comparing specific drug interventions, however, the ACE inhibitor appeared more effective than the other agents in slowing the decline in GFR and proteinuria.[19,20]

SHEP

The Systolic Hypertension in the Elderly Program (SHEP) study included 657 elderly black patients with systolic hypertension, representing 14% of the total.[21] The evaluation was efficacy of chlorthalidone versus placebo in reducing stroke as a primary outcome. Stroke was reduced in black women by 36% but not in black men. Cardiovascular events were reduced by 50% on the basis of unpublished results by SHEP investigators.[21]

Several meta-analyses of antihypertensive drug efficacy in blacks have been published. In an analysis of 15 studies involving 2,902 black subjects and 9,307 white subjects between 1984 and 1998, the percentages of whites/blacks with similar drug-associated changes in diastolic pressure were 90% each for diuretics and β-blockers, 95% for CCBs, and only 81% for ACE inhibitors.[22] For systolic blood pressures, similar blood pressure-associated changes ranged from 83% to 93%. ACE inhibitors and β-blockers resulted in larger blood pressure decreases in whites than in blacks and the opposite was the case with diuretics and CCBs. The results of this analysis suggested to the authors that although modest racial differences in the efficacy of drug classes exist, clinical decisions on drug use may more properly be based on cost, compelling indications, and underlying organ system disease rather than on race.

Another systematic review that evaluated 30 studies of antihypertensive drug therapy in black patients through March 2004[21] can be summarized as follows: (1) most of the antihypertensive drugs were more effective than placebo in reducing systolic and diastolic blood pressure; (2) β-blockers did not differ significantly from placebo in reduction of systolic blood pressure; (3) ACE inhibitors did not differ significantly from placebo in decreasing diastolic blood pressure, but only 23% of actively treated patients in these studies reached target blood pressure goals; and (4) CCBs were the only drug class effective for all subgroups of black participants. The studies' reviewers concluded that although drugs differed in their efficacy of reducing blood pressure, there was no significant difference in morbidity and mortality outcomes if blood pressure reduction goals were achieved.

The efficacy of agents affecting the renin-angiotensin system has generally been less pronounced in blacks than in whites. For example, in patients with left ventricular (LV) dysfunction, enalapril (Vasotec®) has been shown to significantly reduce the risk of hospitalization for white patients with heart failure, but not for blacks.[23] This is especially important in LV dysfunction patients with hypertension However, the selective aldosterone blocker eplerenone (Inspra®) appears to be superior in antihypertensive effects in blacks compared to the ARB losartan (Cozaar®).[24] Eplerenone as well as losartan significantly reduced urinary albumin/creatinine ratios in blacks and whites.

A consensus statement has been published on management of high blood pressure in blacks that uses the results of population-based studies and clinical trials to guide antihypertensive therapy.[25] Most of the recommendations for risk assessment apply to all special groups. A salient feature of risk assessment in blacks emphasizes evidence for renal disease, which is three to four times more likely to lead to ESRD in blacks than in whites. Evaluation should include evidence for albuminuria, with special effort to get blood pressure targets to <130/80 mm Hg with nondiabetic renal disease and albuminuria of >1 g/day. Summaries of the use of antihypertensive agents and management issues in blacks are found in Tables 4-2 and 4-3.

In terms of lifestyle modification, salt (sodium) restriction appears to lead to more pronounced blood pressure lowering in blacks than in other groups.[26] The greater salt sensitivity in blacks may also be associated with lower potassium intake than in whites, so that potassium intakes should also be emphasized in the absence of renal failure.

The evaluation of pharmacologic intervention points out that all classes of antihypertensive agents will lower blood pressure in blacks, but that the blood pressure-lowering efficacy of thiazide diuretics and dihydropyridine CCBs are particularly effective, in comparison with ACE inhibitors, ARBs, or β-blockers. However, most patients need two

Table 4-2: Considerations Regarding the Use of Antihypertensive Classes in African-American Patients With High Blood Pressure

Class	Potential Disadvantages
Diuretics Thiazide diuretics	High doses should be avoided Potential for erectile dysfunction Potential for hypokalemia, particularly if sodium is not restricted Minimal efficacy with decreasing GFR (eg, GFR <45 mL/min per 1.73m^2)
Potassium-sparing diuretics	Observe for hyperkalemia

ACE=Angiotensin-converting enzyme, ALLHAT= Antihypertensive and Lipid-Lowering treatment to prevent Heart Attack Trial, ARB=angiotensin II receptor blocker, CHD=coronary heart disease, GFR=glomerular filtration rate, ISH=isolated systolic hypertension

Potential Benefits

Inexpensive and well tolerated

Efficacy and reduction of stroke and CHD events demonstrated in elderly, African Americans, ISH, and heart failure patients

Low-dose thiazide diuretics (eg, hydrochlorothiazide 12.5-25 mg/d) potentiate the blood pressure-lowering effects of other classes of agents, including ACE inhibitors, ARBs, and β-blockers

Patients at risk of hypokalemia

Potential benefits in heart failure

Data Regarding Use in African Americans*

Efficacy for use in low-dose combination therapy well established for African Americans

Chlorthalidone demonstrated cardiovascular (CV) benefits for African Americans in ALLHAT

Recent evidence (for blood-pressure-lowering efficacy) with a selective aldosterone blocker (eplerenone) in African Americans

*Contrasts in efficacy for African Americans should be viewed with caution, since they have not been established in randomized controlled trials.

(continued on next page)

Table 4-2: Considerations Regarding the Use of Antihypertensive Classes in African-American Patients With High Blood Pressure (continued)

Class	Potential Disadvantages
Loop diuretics	Must be taken 2-3 times/d to control volume
	Risk of hypovolemia or hypokalemia
	Should not be used in patients with normal kidney function
β-Blockers	Cautious use in patients with reactive airway diseases or depression
α-Antagonists	No evidence for CV benefits
	Risk of postural hypotension

Potential Benefits	**Data Regarding Use in African Americans**
Reserved for use in patients with renal insufficiency (serum creatinine >2.0 mg/dL [>177 μmol/L] for men and >1-8 mg/dL [>159 μmol/L for women])	Not available
Indicated for post-MI	Evidence of benefits in African-American patients post-MI
	Evidence of less blood-pressure-lowering efficacy as monotherapy in African-American vs white patients
Indicated for benign prostatic hypertrophy	Negative data reported in ALLHAT for doxazosin in African-American patients

MI=myocardial infarction

(continued on next page)

Table 4-2: Considerations Regarding the Use of Antihypertensive Classes in African-American Patients With High Blood Pressure *(continued)*

Class	Potential Disadvantages
CCBs	Rapid- or short-acting CCBs contraindicated
	Dihydropyridine CCBs: potential for pedal edema. Observe for hyperkalemia, particularly at higher doses
	Nondihydropyridine CCBs: potential for conduction abnormalities, constipation: consider potential drug-drug interactions
ACE Inhibitors	Adverse effect of bothersome dry cough in some patients
	Angioedema (rare)

CCB=calcium channel blocker

Potential Benefits

Dihydropyridine CCBs are potent vasodilators possessing high efficacy at reducing blood pressure

CCBs reduce stroke and CV events in a wide range of patients

High tolerability

Indicated for prevention of CV events and for target-organ protection in patients with diabetes, heart failure, post-MI, diabetic nephropathy

Data Regarding Use in African Americans

Evidence of efficacy and benefits in African-American patients is well established

Some evidence of renal benefits in African-American patients

AASK found that a dihydropyridine CCB (amlodipine) was less renoprotective than ACE inhibitors in African-American patients with hypertensive renal insufficiency

Strong evidence of target organ protection in African-American patients

In AASK, some evidence of less blood pressure-lowering efficacy as monotherapy in African-American vs white patients

Some evidence of more cough and angioedema related to ACE inhibitor therapy in African-American patients compared with white patients

(continued on next page)

Table 4-2: Considerations Regarding the Use of Antihypertensive Classes in African-American Patients With High Blood Pressure *(continued)*

Class	Potential Disadvantages
ARBs	Newest class of agents, so less data on clinical outcomes

or more antihypertensive agents to bring blood pressure to target goals, so combinations of agents may mitigate these differences in relative efficacy. In blacks as well as in other groups, low doses of two agents yield additional decreases of blood pressure of 8-11/4-6 mm Hg compared with the highest dose of monotherapy.[27] The importance of ARBs was noted in the AASK trial, in which the ACE inhibitor ramipril (Altace®) reduced clinical events by 46% compared with the dihydropyridine CCB amlodipine, and reduced decline in kidney function to a significantly greater extent than did amlodipine and metoprolol. Angiotensin II receptor blockers have been especially useful in blacks

Potential Benefits

High tolerability

Benefits shown for target-organ protection in patients with diabetic nephropathy of early renal insufficiency

Evidence of benefits for patients with heart failure

Data Regarding Use in African Americans

Small studies show blood pressure-lowering efficacy in African Americans, particularly in combination with hydrochlorothiazide

AASK=African-American Study of Kidney Disease and Hypertension, ACE=Angiotensin-converting enzyme, ARBs=angiotensin II receptor blocker

From Douglas[25] with permission.

when combined with thiazide diuretics, especially in type II diabetic nephropathy. ACE inhibitors are useful in LV dysfunction but blacks appear to be at increased risk for side effects from these agents, such as cough and angio-edema.[28,29]

Hispanics

In the 2003-2004 NHANES survey, Mexican Americans had a similar age-adjusted prevalence of hypertension compared with non-Hispanic whites, approximately 28%. Although there was improvement in hypertension awareness, treatment, and control in non-Hispanic whites and

Table 4-3: Treatment Pearls: Management of High Blood Pressure in African Americans

- Compared with white Americans, African Americans are at greater risk for the development of high blood pressure, type 2 diabetes mellitus, coronary heart disease (CHD), heart failure, left vertricular hypertension, stroke, and end-stage renal disease. These facts suggest the need to obtain blood pressure measurements and assess risk for cardiovascular disease in African Americans at regular intervals across the life span in all primary care settings.

- Clinicians should make concerted efforts to increase awareness among African Americans of the links between lifestyle choices and cardiovascular and renal outcomes.

- Both high dietary sodium and low dietery potassium intake may contribute to excess high blood pressure in African Americans. Clinicians should recommend increasing dietary potassium while moderating sodium intake to the recommended <2.4 g/d.

- Obesity and inactivity are particularly prevalent among African American women and should be viewed as major cardiovascular risk factors in all African Americans.

- The Dietary Approaches to Stop Hypertension (DASH) diet was found to be particularty beneficial in lowering blood pressure in African Americans. Information about this diet is readily available and should be provided to patients.

- African Americans have a high prevalence of type 2 diabetes mellitus. Based on current National Cholesterol Education Program guidelines, patients with type 2 diabetes have a CHD risk that is equivalent to the risk for patients with CHD and require intensive interventions to lower low-density lipoprotein cholesterol levels to the goal of <100 mg/dL (<2.59 mmol/L).

- The perception that it is more medically difficult to lower blood pressure in African Americans than in other patients is unjustified.

- All antihypertensive drug classes are associated with blood pressure-lowering efficacy in African Americans, although combination therapy may frequently be required to achieve and maintain target blood pressure.

- As monotherapy, β-blockers and angiotensin-converting enzyme (ACE) inhibitors may produce less blood pressure-lowering effects in African Americans than in whites.

- Thiazide diuretics and calcium channel blockers may have greater blood pressure-lowering efficacy than do other classes in African Americans.

- Where compelling indications have been identified for prescribing specific classes of agents, such as β-blockers or renin-angiotensin system-blocking agents (ACE inhibitors or angiotensin II receptor blockers), these compelling indications should be applied equally to African American patients.

- When prescribing ACE inhibitors, it is important to note that compared with whites, African Americans appear to be at increased risk for ACE inhibitor-associated angioedema, cough, or both. All patients should be instructed to report any symptoms related to angioedema promptly.

From Douglas[25] with permission.

blacks between NHANES II (1976-1980) and NHANES III (1988-1991), no changes were found between a Hispanic Health and Nutrition survey (1982-1984) and NHANES III in Mexican Americans.[30] Although these disparities between non-Hispanics and Mexican Americans persisted through the 2002 survey, the survey in 2003-2004 demonstrated an improvement of awareness (from 57%-64%), and treatment (from 37%-48%), but still lower than non-Hispanics. Blood pressure control was found to be lowest in Mexican Americans (27%) compared with blacks and non-Hispanic whites. In the ALLHAT study, in which *Hispanic whites* comprised 16% of the total group, an interesting finding was that this racial group, although having less blood pressure control at enrollment, had a higher control at 4 years into the study (72%) than did non-Hispanic whites (67%) and non-Hispanic blacks (59%).[30] This finding suggested that Hispanic ethnicity did not necessarily presage inferior blood pressure control when there was equal access to medical care and when medication cost was not an issue under the auspices of a clinical trial.[30]

In the International Verapamil SR/Trandolapril (INVEST) trial as well, the Hispanic cohort had better blood pressure control and lower risk of adverse cardiovascular outcomes than did the non-Hispanic cohort.[31] The patients were randomized to sustained-release verapamil (with trandolapril) or atenolol (with hydrochlorothiazide). With Hispanic patients grouped together whatever the treatment regimen, the primary outcome of nonfatal MI, nonfatal stroke, or death was lower than that in non-Hispanics (RR 0.87, 95% CI, 0.78-0.97) (Figure 4-3). However, there was a trend for greater development of diabetes in Hispanics receiving atenolol and hydrochlorothiazide. But at baseline only 22% of Hispanic patients had blood pressure controlled despite previous antihypertensive treatment, similar to the findings in the NHANES surveys. The increased risk for diabetes in Hispanics, due possibly to the higher prevalence of overweight and obesity compared with other groups, suggests that, since diuretics and β-blockers may be more likely to produce this adverse outcome, these agents should be used cautiously in overweight Hispanic patients. CCBs and ACE inhibitors, on the other hand, would either have a neutral effect or actually increase insulin sensitivity.

Certain explanations for the findings of the NHANES surveys in relation to Hispanic whites compared with non-Hispanic whites include: (1) less health insurance and less preventive services, and (2) lower use of antihypertensive treatment.[32,33]

The importance of dietary salt restriction in blood pressure control was studied in a group of salt-sensitive black, Hispanic, and non-Hispanic white subjects with hypertension in conjunction with antihypertensive agents.[34] The absolute blood pressure achieved by all racial groups was consistently lowered when salt restriction was combined with an ACE inhibitor or a CCB. In all racial groups, the use of a high versus a low salt diet with the ACE inhibitor showed an enhanced effect on blood pressure reduction compared with the CCB.

Conclusions

Some conclusions about the impact of hypertension on various ethnic groups include the following: The incidence of hypertension, mortality from hypertensive disease, stroke and hypertensive renal disease is higher in blacks than in other groups. Some Hispanic Americans appear to have a lower risk for hypertension but a greater risk for risk factors such as diabetes and hyperlipidemia. A similar association of mortality and income is found in blacks and non-black Hispanics.

In response to antihypertensive therapy, blacks respond less favorably to ACE inhibitors and β-blockers, and more favorably to diuretics and CCBs. There appears to be no such hierarchy in response in non-black Hispanics. However, ethnicity cannot predict the initial response in an individual to any class of antihypertensive agent.

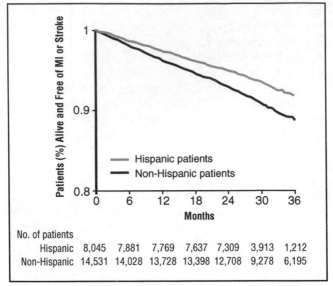

Figure 4-3: From the INVEST trial. An analysis of 8,045 Hispanic patients and 14,351 non-Hispanic patients enrolled. Kaplan-Meier curve of time to primary outcome event of combined nonfatal myocardial infarction, nonfatal stroke, or death, by Hispanic vs non-Hispanic status. From Cooper-DeHoff,[31] with permission.

In terms of clinical trial results of antihypertensive drug therapy, primarily comparing blacks and Hispanics with non-Hispanic whites, several trials showed different clinical outcomes. For example, ALLHAT found a greater magnitude of benefit of diuretics for blacks compared to nonblacks, while the LIFE trial found that ARBs were less effective than β-blockers. Several trials exclusively in Asians have demonstrated CCBs to be effective in preventing cardiovascular outcomes.[35]

Whatever the ethnic minority group, hypertension is not now adequately controlled in the US. Because older persons are a rapidly growing component of the American population, the potential impact of hypertension on the population, in addition to the increased prevalence of diabetes and obesity, becomes even more significant. Although inroads have been made within all racial groups on awareness and treatment of hypertension, efforts at prevention take on increasing importance for decrease in cardiovascular morbidity and mortality. For hypertension prevention, this implies efforts to decrease caloric intake, control the use of salt intake, and increase physical activity. This can only be accomplished within a milieu that encourages the person at risk to modify lifestyle behaviors. Such preventive practices may ultimately serve us better than waiting for blood pressure to increase before intervening with a pharmacologic spectrum. It also makes economic sense.

References

1.   Adams JM: Some racial differences in blood pressure and morbidity in groups of white and colored workmen. *Am J Med Sci* 1932; 184:342.

2.   Hajjar I, Kotcen TA: Trends in prevalence, awareness, treatment, and control of hypertension in the Unites States, 1988-2000. *JAMA* 2003;290:199-206.

3.   Hertz RP, Ungar AN, Cornell JA, et al: Racial disparities in hypertensive prevalence, awareness and management. *Arch Intern Med* 2005;165:2098-2104.

4.   Ong KL, Cheung BMY, Man YB, et al: Prevalence, awareness, treatment and control of hypertension among United States adults 1999-2004. *Hypertension* 2007;49:69-75.

5.   Kramer H, Han C, Post W, et al: Racial/ethnic differences in hypertension and hypertension treatment and control in the multi-ethnic study of atherosclerosis (MESA). *Am J Hypertens* 2004;17:963-970.

6.   Hicks LS, Fairchild DG, Horng MS, et al: Determinants of JNC VI guideline adherence, intensity of drug therapy, and blood pressure control by race and ethnicity. *Hypertension* 2004;44:429-434.

7.   Howard F, Prineas R, Moy C, et al: Racial and geographic differences in awareness, treatment, and control of hypertension. The reasons for geographic and racial differences in stroke study. *Stroke* 2006;37:1171-1178.

8.   Harris MI, Flegal KM, Cowie CC, et al: Prevalence of diabetes, impaired fasting glucose, and impaired glucose tolerance in US adults; the Third National Health and Nutrition Survey, 1988-1994. *Diabetes Care* 1998;21:518-524.

9.   Rehman SU, Hutchison FN, Hendrix K, et al: Ethnic differences in blood pressure control among men at Veterans Affairs clinics and other health care sites. *Arch Intern Med* 2005;165:1041-1047.

10.   Rawaf MM, Kressin NR: Exploring racial and demographic trends in physician behavior, physician trust and their associations with blood pressure control. *J Natl Med Assoc* 2007;99:1248-1254.

11.   Racial/ethnic disparities in prevalence, treatment, and control of hypertension—United States 1999-2002. *MMWR* 2005;54:7-9.

12.   Giles T, Aranda JM Jr, Suh DC, et al: Ethnic/racial variations in blood pressure awareness, treatment, and control. *J Clin Hypertens* 2007; 9:345-354.

13.   Preston RA, Materson BJ, Reda DJ, et al: Age-race subgroup compared with renin profile as predictors of blood pressure response to antihypertensive therapy. Department of Veterans Affairs Cooperative Study Group on Antihypertensive Agents. *JAMA* 1998;280:1168-1172.

14.   Saunders E, Weir MR, Kong BW, et al: A comparison of efficacy and safety of a beta-blocker, a calcium channel blocker, and a converting enzyme inhibitor in hypertensive blacks. *Arch Intern Med* 1990;150:1707-1713.

15.   Major outcomes in high-risk hypertensive patients randomized to angiotensin-converting enzyme inhibitor or calcium channel blocker vs diuretic: The Antihypertensive and Lipid-Lowering treatment to Prevent Heart Attack (ALLHAT). *JAMA* 2002;288:2981-2997.

16.   Wright JT Jr, Dunn JK, Cutler JA, et al: Outcomes in antihypertensive black and non-black patients treated with chlorthalidone, amlodipine, and lisinopril. *JAMA* 2005;293:1595-1608.

17.   Dahlof B, Devereux RB, Kjeldsen SE, et al: Cardiovascular morbidity and mortality in the Losartan Intervention for End-point reduction in hypertension study (LIFE); a randomized trial against atenolol. *Lancet* 2002;359:995-1003.

18.   Julius S, Alderman MH, Beevers G, et al: Cardiovascular risk reduction in hypertensive black patients with left ventricular hypertrophy: the LIFE study. *J Am Coll Cardiol* 2004;43:1047-1055.

19. Wright JT Jr, Bakris G, Greene T, et al: Effect of blood pressure lowering and antihypertensive drug class on progression of hypertensive kidney disease; results from the AASK trial. *JAMA* 2002;288:2421-2431.

20. Agadoa LY, Appel L, Bakris GL, et al: Effect of ramipril vs amlodipine on renal outcomes in hypertensive nephrosclerosis: a randomized controlled trial. *JAMA* 2001;285:2719-2728.

21. Brewster LM, van Montfrans GA, Kleijnen J: Systematic review: antihypertensive drug therapy in black patients. *Ann Intern Med* 2004;141:614-627.

22. Sehgal AR: Overlap between whites and blacks in response to antihypertensive drugs. *Hypertension* 2004;43:566-572.

23. Exner DV, Dries DL, Domanski MJ, Cohn JN: Lesser response of angiotensin-converting-enzyme inhibitor therapy in black as compared with white patients with left ventricular dysfunction. *N Engl J Med* 2001;344:1351-1357.

24. Flack JM, Oparil S, Pratt JH, et al: Efficacy and tolerability of eplerenone and losartan in hypertensive black and white patients. *J Am Coll Cardiol* 2003;41:1148-1155.

25. Douglas JG, Bakris GL, Epstein M, et al: Management of high blood pressure in African Americans: consensus statement of the Hypertension in African American Working Group of the International Society on Hypertension in Blacks. *Arch Intern Med* 2003; 163:525-541.

26. Sacks FM, Svetkey LP, Vollmer WM, et al, for the DASH–Sodium Collaborative Research Group: Effects on blood pressure of reduced dietary sodium and the Dietary Approaches to Hypertension (DASH) diet. *N Engl J Med* 2001;344:3-10.

27. Fogari R, Corea L, Cardoni O, et al: Combined therapy with benazepril and amlodipine in the treatment of hypertension inadequately treated by an ACE inhibitor alone. *J Cardiovasc Pharmacol* 1997;30:443-462.

28. Brown NJ, Ray WA, Snowden M, et al: Black Americans have an increased rate of angiotensin converting enzyme inhibitor-associated angioedema. *Clin Pharmacol Ther* 1996;60:8-13.

29. Elliott WJ: Higher incidence of discontinuation of angiotensin converting enzyme inhibitors due to cough in black subjects. *Clin Pharmacol Ther* 1996;60:582-588.

113

30. Margolis KL, Piller LR, Ford CE, et al: Blood pressure control in Hispanics in the Antihypertensive and Lipid-lowering Treatment to Prevent Heart Attack trial. *Hypertension* 2007;50:854-861.

31. Cooper-DeHoff RM, Aranda JM Jr, Gaxiola E, et al: Blood pressure control and cardiovascular outcomes in high-risk Hispanic patients-findings from the International Verapamil SR/Trandilopril Study (INVEST). *Am Heart J* 2006;151:1072-1079.

32. Centers for Disease Control and Prevention: Access to healthcare and preventive services among Hispanics and non-Hispanics–United States 2001-2002. *MMWR Morbid Mortal Wkly Rep* 2004;53:937-941.

33. Ayala C, Neff LJ, Croft JB, et al: Prevalence of self-reported high blood pressure awareness, advice received from health professionals, and actions taken to reduce high blood pressure among US adults–Healthstyles 2002. *J Clin Hypertens* 2005;7:513-519.

34. Weir MR, Crysant SG, McCarron DA, et al: Influence of race and dietary salt on the antihypertensive efficacy of an angiotensin-converting enzyme inhibitor or a calcium channel antagonist in salt-sensitive hypertensives. *Hypertension* 1998;31:1088-1096.

35. Park IU, Taylor AL: Race and ethnicity in trials of antihypertensive therapy to prevent cardiovascular outcomes: a systematic review. *Ann Fam Med* 2007;5:444-452.

Chapter 5

Diagnosis and Treatment of Coronary Artery Disease

By L. Veronica Lee, MD
and JoAnne Micale Foody, MD

Coronary artery disease (CAD) is the most common cause of death in the United States and kills a higher relative number of African Americans than Caucasians. There is a higher prevalence of the traditional risk factors in African Americans than in Caucasians, but this does not completely explain the overall disparity. African Americans have been found to present earlier with CAD, and have a higher mortality, especially out of hospital, in part from a higher risk of sudden cardiac death and from a higher rate of first myocardial infarction (MI) independent of age.[1] Hispanics, a racially diverse ethnic group, have demonstrated a recent acceleration in both cardiovascular risk as manifested by the increasing prevalence of the metabolic syndrome, and in cardiovascular disease (CVD) mortality. Recent studies have clarified some of the increased risk seen in the Native-American population and the increasing risk in the Asian population that was considered, overall, to be a low-risk group until recent years.

The differences between racial and ethnic groups may be related to a lack of access and information for both the general population and health-care providers, which may delay or underestimate risk. To more fully understand these differences, one needs to look at the tools used to diagnose and treat CAD as well as the social factors involved.

Diagnosis of Coronary Artery Disease

Diagnosis of an acute coronary syndrome (ACS) such as MI and unstable angina (UA) is made using electrocardiogram (ECG) and cardiac enzyme criteria. Electrocardiogram abnormalities are more common in African Americans than in Caucasians, partly as the result of a higher prevalence of left ventricular hypertrophy (LVH) with strain patterns that can mimic an abnormality that would otherwise be diagnostic of an ACS. Some of these differences are the result of a history of untreated hypertension, athletic lifestyle, and/or genetics. The presence of LVH can also reduce the sensitivity of the ECG for detection of active ischemia and MI. There have been no significant differences noted between races in creatine kinase (CK), CK-MB, and troponin I and T assays.

To explore the racial differences in ECG further, Strogatz et al[2] studied a 20-year follow-up of African-American men (164 of 308) and Caucasian (159 of 511) men 40 to 64 years of age with major or minor ECG abnormalities. Those abnormalities were defined by the Pooling project and were associated with increasing age and blood pressure. Findings were adjusted for cardiovascular risk factors, and major ECG abnormalities (ST depression, T-wave inversion, left bundle branch block [LBBB], right bundle branch block [RBBB], atrial flutter, atrioventricular [AV] block, or premature ventricular contractions [PVC]) were found to be associated with an increase in all-cause or cardiovascular mortality in both African Americans (relative risk [RR]=1.7) and Caucasians (RR=2.2). These findings suggest that major ECG abnormalities have a similar predictive value for both races. Strogatz et al also suggest that R-wave voltage indicative of LVH may be less important than the presence of hypertension causing the elevations.

Left ventricular hypertrophy is associated with increased cardiovascular morbidity and mortality in hypertensive patients.[3-5] Although African Americans are known to have more baseline ECG abnormalities, current ECG criteria are not as specific for African Americans as for Caucasians.[6-13] Although LVH is associated with increased cardiovascular events, this may not be the case for African Americans who have greater ECG LVH diagnosed, out of proportion to both blood pressure and echocardiographic findings. Echocardiography has, in fact, found only minor differences in quantifiable left ventricular (LV) chamber size, LV mass, and LVH between Caucasians and African Americans, which are far less than those diagnosed by ECG criteria.[14-18] To explore this further, the Losartan Intervention for Endpoint Reduction in Hypertension (LIFE) trial enrolled patients with hypertension and LVH by either the Cornell voltage–duration product or Sokolow-Lyon voltage criteria and were treated in a double-blind antihypertensive regimen with losartan and atenolol.[19] Echocardiography was performed in 871 patients (751 Caucasians and 120 African Americans). The study found that the diagnosis of LVH by ECG criteria using voltage and voltage-duration product criteria is related to ethnicity and not echocardiographic LVH. Differences were not associated with increased LV mass, or body mass index (BMI). The QRS area is a better measure for LVH, which takes into account the narrower QRS and taller complex typically seen in African Americans.

Another study that emphasizes the differences in ECG found in healthy members of different races is one of elite US football players. This study demonstrated significant ECG differences between African-American and Caucasian players.[20] Abnormal ECG findings were present in 25% of 480 players (30% African American n=396, 13% Caucasian n=78, P <0.0001; risk ratio after multivariable adjustment [RR] 2.03, 95% confidence interval [CI] 1.56-2.64, P <0.0001), and abnormal ECGs consistent with a diagnosis of CAD were more common in African Americans (n=76, 6%) than in Caucasians (n=11, 2%; RR 2.59, 95% CI, 1.18 to 5.67, P <0.02). Abnormal ECGs were also related to player position, especially wide receivers (n=91; 35%). Ten percent of players received ECGs, which did not show structural abnormalities. Even in athletes there appear to be significant racial differences in ECGs and the abnormalities that may confound interpretation of active CAD.

Less is known about other races and ethnic groups in regard to ECG. The Strong Heart Study (SHS) reported that there was an association in Native Americans with diabetes with ECG repolarization abnormalities and all-cause CVD mortality.[21] ST segment depression was associated with a 3.68 increase in risk compared to participants without an ST abnormality after adjustment for glucose and other cardiac risk factors. In addition, SHS demonstrated an additive increase in 3-year mortality when the finding of LVH diagnosed by ECG was present with ST segment depression on ECG.[22]

A prospective study assessed ECG abnormalities (arrhythmias, RBBB, LBBB, AV conduction delays, and LVH) with CVD death and morbidity in 1,605 diabetic Pima Indians at least 35 years of age.[23] The determined hazard ratio adjusting for confounding variables (traditional cardiac risk factors and proteinuria) and participants with minor and major ischemic ECG abnormalities had a 1.22-fold (95% CI, 0.76-1.97) and 1.83-fold (95% CI, 1.21-2.76) greater CVD mortality, and 1.32-fold (95% CI, 0.70-2.50) and 2.12-fold (95% CI, 1.26-3.57) increase in CAD death rate compared to those without ischemic ECG changes, respectively.

The ECG is a major component of our ability to detect, diagnose, and follow CAD; however, there is still limited information pertaining to it about differences in key racial and ethnic groups. In addition, as seen in African Americans, standard criteria overdiagnose LVH, and allowances are not made for this lack of specificity and the reduced sensitivity in the presence of baseline ECG abnormalities for ongoing ischemia. Future studies will need to study how to accurately use ECG information in a racially specific way to improve diagnosis.

Stress Testing

The differences in ECG become important in stress testing because it is the mainstay of the diagnosis of CAD in patients with chest discomfort or for those who are at risk of CAD. Treadmill ECG testing can lack the specificity and sensitivity in people with baseline abnormalities from LVH. In addition, nuclear imaging used to assist in the assessment of patients with baseline abnormalities in ECG has only been assessed in a limited fashion for racial and ethnic differences. One study assessed 1,086 Caucasian and African-American patients with known or suspected CAD and stress testing performed with technetium-99m imaging by all-cause mortality over 24 months.[24] Overall mortality was not predicted by normal stress testing in African Americans (all-cause death 2.8× more common than in Caucasians) although this group had a lower risk of cardiovascular events than did the Caucasians with normal studies. The study did not determine the etiology of the noncardiac causes of death, and there was only a total of 26 events in the African-American group. Abnormal studies in both African Americans and Caucasians correlated with a higher cardiovascular event rate. In the presence of hypertensive heart disease, the false-positive rate may be higher in the African-American population.

Other racial and ethnic differences are noted in the use of stress testing in suspected CAD. Stress testing is an important determinant for decisions about prevention and more invasive therapy for these patients. There are observed differences in the use of diagnostic stress testing in the African-American population, which was further assessed in a prospective case-control study of patients on Medicare, who had similar access to medical care, and who were at least 66 years of age. It is known that African Americans are more often uninsured or underinsured, and may refuse more invasive therapy for CAD.[25-32] African-American men were less likely to receive stress testing compared to Caucasian men with similar cardiac risk factor profiles, and this was not related to the number of physician visits. This small study could not determine whether the reduced amount of stress testing in African Americans increased the CVD event rate, or if there was relative over-testing in the Caucasian male group. Further study will be needed to assess this. Interestingly, a population-based study of Medicare recipients from 1993 to 2001 showed a general increase in the use of stress testing, cardiac catheterization, and percutaneous transluminal coronary recanalization (PTCR), but racial differences in utilization of these procedures persisted over time.[33] It is unclear whether this represents underutilization in some groups and/or an overutilization in other groups.

Preoperative evaluation relies heavily on the use of stress testing in selected patients. To assess racial disparities in stress test performance as part of a preoperative evaluation, a study evaluated 314 patients with stable, known CAD for noncardiac surgery and general anesthesia.[34] Of the patients enrolled, 222 were evaluable and 23% were African American. Previous studies have suggested that there is a high refusal rate of African Americans for elective catheterization after an abnormal stress test (32% African American and 17% Caucasian) as opposed to post MI. Some of the reasons for this may be lack of trust, lack of familiarity with testing, and religious beliefs.[35,36] In this study, the refusal rate was <5% for testing. There was no difference in use of stress testing, ECGs, and Holter monitors. A lower use of catheterization was seen in the African-American population (8.7% vs 50% Caucasian, P=0.0001), but when corrected for the higher prevalence of ischemic cardiomyopathy in Caucasians (2.64-fold higher) and presence of CAD, race did not appear to predict underuse of cardiac catheterization. No racial differences were found in mortality and morbidity in this small study.

An alternative to nuclear stress testing is echocardiography performed with either an exercise treadmill or dobutamine. A study looked at the hemodynamic effects of dobutamine in 150 patients (African American=26).[37] Hypertension, chest pain, arrhythmia, and nausea occurred in 19.2% of African Americans compared to 8% of Caucasians (P=0.08). African-American patients also had significantly higher blood pressure at all doses of dobutamine compared to Caucasians, which was partly explained by a higher baseline blood pressure in African-American patients. No difference was found in chronotropic response in this small study. The investigator concluded that because of a higher termination rate in African Americans because of a hypertensive response to dobutamine, this form of testing might not be optimal for this group.

Additional Imaging: Echocardiography and Calcium Scoring

Unlike ECG, echocardiography does not routinely adjust for race or ethnicity in defining normal values. A study that raises the importance of considering this is a substudy of the SHS, which assessed 1,457 participants from Arizona, Oklahoma, and North/South Dakota without a prior diagnosis of CAD or diabetes mellitus by echocardiography. At baseline the participants from Arizona had lower heart rates and the highest BMI. Echo measurements revealed more LVH in the Arizona (23%, concentric pattern predominates) and the Dakotas (18%, eccentric pattern predominates) groups compared to the Oklahoma group (15%; P=0.01) and were independent of heart rate, BMI, blood pressure, and glucose tolerance testing. There was no significant difference in fractional shortening or ejection fraction. Left ventricular midwall shortening with and without stress correction has been found to be an independent predictor of major cardiovascular events in hypertensive patients who are asymptomatic.[38] The Arizona cohort that had a higher cardiovascular event rate also had abnormally low contractility using these measures (9.9% compared to 6.4% Dakotas and 6.6% Oklahoma; P=0.03).[39,40] This difference was independent of heart rate, blood pressure, BMI, and abnormal glucose tolerance testing. In parallel to the overall lower blood pressure, increased LV chamber size and lesser LV wall thickness of the Dakota participants, is a higher relative cardiac output and lower peripheral resistance. These findings were independent of other risk factors and may represent differences in lifestyle or genetics. These differences within a single racial group emphasize the importance of genetic variability in understanding the differences in presentation of disease in different racial and ethnic groups, since these groups may be far more diverse than the present groups studied.

Mitral annular calcification (MAC) is a finding on echocardiography of calcium deposits at the level of the mitral annulus and has been found to correlate with increased age (>70 yr), female gender, and renal disease in Caucasian populations. Several studies, including the Framingham Heart Study, have found the presence of MAC to be a risk factor for CHD events, as well as for stroke and congestive heart failure (CHF).[41-51] The Atherosclerosis Risk in Communities (ARIC) investigators found that MAC in the African-American population was a significant risk factor for CVD events (fatal and nonfatal MI and revascularization) in 2,409 African Americans with a hazard ratio (HR)=2.32 (95% CI, 1.11-4.87). Hispanics also have an increased risk of CVD events with the presence of MAC. They had a similar risk profile to Caucasians with MAC, which was more prominent in women, smokers, and people with multiple traditional cardiac risk factors.[52] This has not been evaluated in other ethnic and racial groups.

Calcification has become an important marker for CVD. not only presenting as MAC, but also in the coronary arteries. Coronary artery calcification (CAC) scoring, using electron beam tomography, is a marker for the presence of angiographic disease from atherosclerosis. Decreased prevalence of CAC is seen in different ethnic groups, but the presence of an abnormal score still correlates with the presence of CAD. In the Multi-Ethnic Study of Atherosclerosis (MESA) population-based study, including 6,000 participants without known CAD or diabetes treatment,[53-55] CAC scores were highest in Caucasian men—70% versus 52% in African-American men, 56% in Hispanic-American men, and 59% in Asian men.[55] Women in general had lower scores (45% Caucasian, 37% African American, 35% Hispanic American, and 42% Asian). Increase in CAC is related to age and male gender, especially in Caucasian and Hispanic-American men.[54] In addition, after adjustment for age, gender, and income, and control for concomitant risk factors (BMI, smoking, diabetes mellitus, hypertension, lipids), birth outside of the US demonstrated lower CAC scores for both African Americans and Hispanic Americans. Asians (Chinese) demonstrated an increase in CAC with a greater duration of living in the US. Fewer years of education completed correlated with higher CAC scores in Caucasians and lower scores in Hispanic Americans.

One study assessed racial and ethnic calcium scoring differences in men and women using 16,560 asymptomatic subjects referred for calcium artery scoring, of which 610 were African American, 1,336 Asian, and 1,256 Hispanic American.[56] The study had findings similar to the MESA population-based study and determined that Caucasians and Hispanic Americans had similar degrees of calcification, whereas African Americans and Asians had less calcium, even with adjustment for cardiac risk factors. When gender was also evaluated, African-American women were more likely to have elevated calcium scores compared to other women. This could potentially be the result of differences in degree of atherosclerosis or differences in the mechanism of significant CAD. A recent study found that

East-Asian women had a trend toward higher CAC scores compared with other women.[57] Unlike MESA, which only studied Chinese women, the difference may be the result of broader cultural and ethnic differences. What is significant is that this overall lower-risk group would have higher CAC scores.

Several new imaging modalities are available for determining the presence of CAD and quantifying its severity. These include magnetic resonance imaging (MRI) with and without angiography, computed tomography (CT) angiography, and positron emission tomography (PET), all of which have yet to be assessed in different ethnic and racial populations. In the future their use in risk stratification and diagnosis will be clarified.

Treatment of Coronary Artery Disease
Bystander Cardiopulmonary Resuscitation

Acute coronary syndrome treatment starts before a patient arrives at the emergency department. Bystander cardiopulmonary resuscitation (CPR), out of hospital, is a critical link in the American Heart Association (AHA) Chain of Survival. Out-of-hospital cardiac arrest has been shown to be delivered less to African-American patients than to Caucasians, with roughly twice as many Caucasians receiving bystander CPR.[58-60] Differences in CPR in 1,379 consecutive non-Hispanic-American and Hispanic-American patients with an out-of-hospital cardiac arrest were evaluated in one study.[61] Of note, 952 were excluded from analysis because race and ethnicity were not documented. This study found that Hispanic Americans were less likely to receive bystander CPR (32.2% vs 41.5% non-Hispanic American; P <0.0001). Hispanic Americans tended to be younger and more often presented with asystole. No survival difference to hospital discharge was found, but this may be due in part to the younger age of Hispanic Americans. Frequently, a family member performs CPR, so some of the racial disparity may result from a lack of training or limited access to CPR classes by African Americans and Hispanic Americans.

Presentation of CAD

Symptoms on presentation are different between Caucasian men, who present with the more classic chest pressure, and African Americans and women, who present with more atypical symptoms.[62] There is a delay in obtaining ECG in African-American patients presenting with chest pain.[63] There is a clear delay in presentation of African Americans for treatment of ACS—as much as three times longer than for Caucasians.[64-67] Some of the delay may be the result of a lack of access to medical care, lack of education regarding symptoms and CAD, lack of confidence in medical therapy and in the community, and different belief systems. Because African Americans present later and are at higher risk, urgent evaluation and treatment should be performed, but the suspicion of ACS for these patients is lower than for Caucasians, with triage ECGs being performed later and enzyme testing and other noninvasive testing less often.[68-71]

On presentation, Caucasians have more ST-segment elevation MI (STEMI), and African Americans are more likely to present with sudden death, NSTEMI, and UA.[72,73] African Americans have more comorbid risk factors such as hypertension, diabetes, renal insufficiency, smoking, and prior history of heart failure. Correction for these baseline characteristics demonstrates that fewer African-American patients with ACS receive diagnostic catheterization, revascularization, or thrombolysis. If an invasive strategy is performed, as reported in women, African Americans have less obstructive CAD. Since there is a higher rate in African Americans of sudden death, it is likely that some of the <50% nonobstructive narrowing of the coronary arteries is responsible.[74]

Less is known about Hispanic Americans and the so-called "Hispanic paradox." Although Hispanic Americans have a worse cardiac risk factor profile (central obesity, increased BMI, dyslipidemia, smoking, diabetes, less access to care and insurance) than do Caucasians, they appear to have fewer events and decreased mortality.[75] However, small, more focused studies on populations, such as the Corpus Christi Heart Project, found a greater admission rate of Hispanic Americans for CAD than for Caucasians.[76] Part of this may be the result of a lack of data on cardiac sudden death in this population, and a lack of accurate statistics on a partially immigrant population, as well as complexities of accurate data collection because of language barriers and accurate ethnic identification of Hispanic Americans. More data are known about the Mexican-American group in terms of CAD, but this is still limited. The National Health Interview Survey (NHIS) may have had significant underreporting because of language, immigrant status, and other unforeseen barriers.[77] This lower response rate has been seen in other large surveys. The National Death Index, which was used in this study, has a significant reduction in accuracy from Caucasian (>97%) to non-Caucasian (86%). Many Hispanic Americans do not have a Social Security number, and often use mother and father or husband and family surnames.[78] In addition, many of them return to their native country once they are sick and unable to work.[79,80] This study was underpowered to assess CAD risk in the Hispanic-American population. Another reason for the putative "Hispanic paradox" may be the effects of obesity on the development of metabolic syndrome, diabetes, and frank cardiovascular disease.

Cardiac Catheterization and Percutaneous Revascularization

Multiple studies have shown that there is a disparity in the use of cardiac catheterization and PTCR in African Americans compared to Caucasians, although there is a higher incidence of traditional cardiac risk factors in the

African-American population and they achieve similar benefit to therapy with PTCR.[81-85] The ARIC study examined 11,242 patients (mean age 61 years, 22% African American, 43% women) in the use of echocardiography, stress testing, right heart catheterization, and angiography. African Americans without a history of MI were less likely than Caucasians to have an angiogram (0.26, 0.20-0.33; P <0.05), but this disparity improved if there was a known history of MI (0.50, 0.40-0.65; P <0.05). Adjusted mortality rates were higher in African Americans until adjusted for catheterization (interaction P <0.0001 for angiography and history of MI). The findings of this study suggest a perceived lower risk in the African-American group for MI on presentation to the hospital, resulting in underuse of cardiac catheterization in this group.

A recent study explored these differences further in 11,829 consecutive patients (89% Caucasian and 11% African American) who received PTCR for stable or unstable angina and were followed for 1 year.[86] A higher relative percentage of African Americans were women with more comorbid risk factors such as hypertension, chronic renal insufficiency, and diabetes. Caucasians were more likely to smoke, have a family history, dyslipidemia, and/or increased BMI. There was no difference in the indication or response to PTCR between groups. Angiogram findings showed a greater proportion of left anterior descending artery disease in African Americans, and more Caucasians had left main (2.6% African American vs 3.6% Caucasian; P=0.016) and three vessel disease (16.9% vs 20.9%; P <0.001), restenosis of a previously treated vessel, and history of coronary artery bypass graft (CABG). Interestingly, glycoprotein IIb/IIIa inhibitors were used more in African Americans (13.2% vs 9.4%; 9.8% of total population). This could point to a possible use of this therapy as a bridge to PTCR and delay of treatment, but this study did not assess time to procedure in this cohort. African-American race was not found to be a predictor of adverse outcome, in hospital, once baseline differences were controlled. This is consistent with other studies that did not show any short-term racial differences.[87-89] However, mortality at 1-year follow-up was 50% higher in African Americans (9.8% African American vs 6.4% Caucasian, P <0.001). This translated to a relative risk of 1.52 (95% CI [1.22-1.89], P <0.001). Using a Cox regression model, the investigators found that race was an independent predictor of mortality at 1-year from major adverse cardiac events (HR=1.35, 95% CI=1.06-1.71; P=0.01). This mortality difference became greater over time, and revascularization for clinical or angiographic restenosis occurred less in African Americans (13.2% vs 16.4% Caucasian; P=0.02). This was also seen in a recent study at 5-year follow-up of 730 (67% African American) patients treated in Detroit, Michigan, where the survival rate was 41% African American vs. 54% Caucasian (log rank P <0.01). Even after adjustment for comorbid conditions, race remained a significant predictor of major adverse cardiac outcome (death, MI, CHF) with an HR of 1.62 (95% CI=1.01-1.28; P <0.04).[90] Patients in this study received newer PTCR methods and African Americans were a significant proportion of the study population, unlike earlier studies that had not seen a significant difference by race.

The Superior Yield of the New Strategy of Enoxaparin, Revascularization, and Glycoprotein IIa/IIIb Inhibitors (SYNERGY) study evaluated patients with NSTEMI and the benefit they received from treatment with low molecular weight heparin and GP2b3a receptor inhibitors.[91] In this multicenter, randomized, controlled trial there was less use of PTCR (46% Caucasian, 41% African American, and 45% Hispanic American, overall P <0.046) and CABG (20% Caucasian, 16% African American, and 22% Hispanic American, overall P <0.044). This translated into a reduction in mortality and reinfarctions at 30 days of 14% Caucasian, 10% African American, and 14% Hispanic American (overall P <0.034), with no racial differences by 6 months. African Americans had less obstructive CAD than Caucasians on angiography (P <0.0001). The lack of significant angiographic disease is similar to findings of the Global Unstable Angina Registry and Treatment Evaluation (GUARANTEE) Registry.[92] There was evidence that event rates were increasing in the African-American group, with increasing time from hospital discharge. There may be less of a difference seen in the patients treated in this study because of the increased screening and follow-up that patients have during participation in a trial.

Leborgne et al[86] noted in their study that some of the racial differences could be the result of more comorbid risk factors in the African-American population as found in other studies and the presence of an increased proportion of older African-American women in the present study.[93-95] This may reflect the previous findings that African Americans are referred less for angiography and PTCR.[96] On presentation, fewer African Americans in this study had prior CABG or PTCR, giving emphasis to the prior finding that revascularization may be underutilized or that there is a difference in mechanism that underlies presentation in the African-American population.[92] This is suggested by the lower ejection fractions seen on presentation in the African-American population with concomitant diabetes and hypertension, which may result in more microvascular disease not amenable to current methods of revascularization.[97,98] The worse survival rates indicate that postrevascularization, over time, may reflect the presence of concomitant diabetes, hypertension, and the natural progression of the small vessel disease, as well as a lack of medical access for aggressive secondary prevention.

Jacobi et al published a single-center, retrospective, longitudinal cohort study in STEMI patients receiving PTCR and followed them for 1 year. The study did not show any difference in clinical outcome in non-Caucasian patients (67%; N=234, Caucasian n=77, African American n=58, Hispanic American n=81, and Asian n=18).[99] This study had a significant number of non-Caucasian patients compared to other studies, although race and ethnicity were self-reported. In an environment that typically cares for a mixed population, perhaps some of the access and patient-physician follow-up care are improved. This was not assessed in this study; however, there are data to support this in a study of African Americans and Hispanic Americans in New York City, where decreases in all-cause mortality were seen in areas with higher densities of a particular racial group.[100]

Barnhart et al assessed both PTCR and CABG revascularization procedures in the New York State Department of Health Statewide Planning and Research Cooperate System (SPARCS) in 12,555 patients admitted with acute MI in 1996.[101] The highest revascularization rates were seen in Caucasians, 25.8% and Hispanic Americans, 25.2%, compared with African Americans, 15.8% (P <0.001). Caucasians who did not receive revascularization were less like to survive to hospital discharge than were nonrevascularized African Americans or Hispanic Americans. If revascularized, there were no differences in mortality during hospitalization.

Coronary Artery Bypass Surgery

The use of cardiac catheterization increased by 342% in the past 25 years, and 1.26 million PTCRs and 261,000 CABGs were performed in the US in 2005.[102] However, like other invasive treatment, data still show that fewer non-Caucasians receive CABG[96,103,104] and have a higher operative mortality.[105,106] Prior studies have suggested that African Americans are less likely to use hospitals with more board-certified physicians, more subspecialties, more evidence-based management, and newer technologies. A future investigation of the hospital and provider dynamics in CABG mortality in hospitals of different patient operative volume should be performed.

The California CABG outcomes reporting program collected data from 121 hospitals in 2003 and 21,272 CABG patients (Caucasian n=15,069, Hispanic American n=2,561, Asians n=1,772, African American n=785).[107] Non-Caucasian patients were more likely to have hypertension, diabetes mellitus, and chronic renal insufficiency (CRI), and be female, younger, and living with liver disease ($P < 0.05$ for each factor). African Americans had a higher BMI, more heart failure and peripheral arterial disease (PAD) than Caucasians. Hispanic Americans had more heart failure than Caucasians and Asians and had a lower BMI. Observed operative mortality showed no statistically significant variation between races, although there was a trend for Asians to have a higher mortality than Caucasians (3.5% vs 2.8%, $P=0.077$) even though the preoperative mortality predictions were higher for African Americans, Hispanic Americans, and Asians compared to Caucasians.

The University Health System Consortium analyzed 71,949 CABG patients from 2002 to 2005 to assess if higher-volume hospitals demonstrated a reduction in mortality risk for African Americans compared to Caucasians. In-hospital mortality for CABG was 2.0% for Caucasians and 2.8% for African Americans. There was a significant benefit for African Americans and a modest improvement for Caucasians at higher-volume hospitals in terms of in-hospital mortality (race by volume interaction; $P < 0.033$). The greatest difference in racial mortality was seen at very-low-volume hospitals, especially in the South and Midwest (region by volume interaction, $P < 0.033$).

Secondary Prevention:
Post-Acute Coronary Syndrome

In recent decades there has been a 25% reduction in cardiovascular mortality in the US in large part due to prevention. It has been well established that medical therapy with aspirin, angiotensin-converting enzyme (ACE) inhibitors, β-blockers, and HMG Co-A reductase inhib-

131

itors (statins); in addition, lifestyle modifications, such as smoking cessation, have resulted in substantial reduction in serious cardiac adverse events. A recent study assessed the racial differences in post-MI secondary prevention, using data from the National Heart Failure and National Acute Myocardial Infarction Projects of the Centers for Medicaid and Medicare Services (CMS). These projects have a mission to assess and improve quality of care for hospitalized Medicare participants with CHF and acute MI.[108] Using ICD-9 codes, 35,407 cases of acute MI (51.3% men, 48.7% women, 87.3% Caucasian, 7.3% African American, and 4.1% Hispanic American) were evaluated. Evaluation consisted of initial use and prescription at discharge of aspirin, ACE inhibitors, and β-blockers, as well as documented smoking-cessation counseling. Aspirin was given at the rate of 75% to 86% and a β-blocker was given at a rate of 55% to 73% at hospital admission and 61% to 83.5% at hospital discharge in patient subgroups. African-American and Hispanic-American patients were found to be prescribed aspirin and β-blockers less than Caucasians, and this was particularly notable in the Hispanic-American group with either end-stage renal disease (ESRD) or diabetes mellitus. Hispanic-American women were found to receive all medications less than any other group. Smoking cessation counseling was significantly lower in African Americans (29.8%) and Hispanic Americans (32.8%) compared to Caucasians (40.8%). Particularly concerning were the even lower rates of smoking-cessation counseling in Hispanic Americans with diabetes mellitus (13.7%) and in African Americans with diabetes mellitus (16.4%).

A recently published study followed 499 patients with suspected CAD (24% non-Caucasian) and 357 with documented CAD (28% non-Caucasian) who underwent angiography.[109] Similar prescribing practices were found between racial groups for antiplatelet, β-blocker, HMG-CoA reductase inhibitors, and ACE inhibitors (or angiotensin II receptor blockers [ARBs]). It is clear that future investigation needs to be done on how to improve both primary and secondary prevention in non-Caucasian patients.

Putative Mechanistic Differences in CAD

Arterial stiffness is considered a risk factor for cardiovascular disease because of the reduced ability to dilate to local factors such as nitric oxide. It is known to be associated with the presence of concomitant risk factors such as hypertension and diabetes, as well as the presence of atherosclerosis. In a small substudy of ARIC, stiffness was assessed in 268 African Americans and 2,459 Caucasians, 45 to 64 years of age, without a prior diagnosis of CHD, computer-aided ventilation (CAV), or transient ischemic attack (TIA).[110] The investigators concluded, using brachial blood pressure and carotid ultrasound, that either stiffness occurred earlier in African Americans or was more accelerated in African Americans compared to Caucasians. This study, unlike earlier ones, controlled for confounding factors such as hypertension, but racial differences, though blunted, persisted with this strategy. This study suggests the importance of early aggressive therapy in African Americans to prevent the effects of comorbidities as well as as-yet-unidentified causes of increased arterial stiffness in African Americans.

In addition, hypertension and diabetes through insulin resistance can result in LVH and other structural abnormalities that predispose patients to increased mortality from CAD. There appears to be a racial dichotomy, as detailed in one study comparing Caucasian Europeans with African Caribbeans in 1,166 patients with left ventricular structure assessed in terms of LVH. Throughout the range of glucose intolerance to frank diabetes, the African Caribbeans had a greater degree of LVH, interventricular septal thickness, and left ventricular mass index, although the investigators suggested that this was the result of higher blood pressure at baseline in this group compared to Europeans.[111]

Endothelial dysfunction is associated with increased cardiovascular events. A study using the precursor of nitric oxide, L-arginine, as an intracoronary infusion showed a greater increase in endothelium-dependent vascular relaxation after acetylcholine stimulation in the African-American cohort as opposed to Caucasians.[112] A placebo arm was not performed; however, this suggests a potentially significant and treatable mechanism for small vessel disease that appears to be more prominent in the African-American population. Another marker of endothelial function, endothelin-1, is greater in African Americans with hypertension than in Caucasians with hypertension, which could stimulate a greater response in vasoconstriction, plaque rupture, and, over time, LVH.[113]

Inflammatory markers, such as C-reactive protein and fibrinogen concentration, tend to be higher in African Americans than in Caucasians; whether or not this is the result of a higher incidence of comorbid conditions such as asthma has yet to be determined.[114,115] In addition, fibrinolytic activity is higher in the African-American population, suggesting a reduced procoagulable state compared to Caucasians.

References

1.   Clark LT: Issues in minority health: atherosclerosis and coronary heart disease in African Americans. *Med Clin N Am* 2005;89: 977-1001.

2.   Strogatz DS, Tyroler HA, Watkins L, et al: Electrocardiographic abnormalities and mortality among middle-aged black men and white men of Evans County, Georgia. *J Chronic Dis* 1987; 40(2):149-155.

3.   Levy D, Garrison RJ, Savage DD, et al: Prognostic implications of echocardiographically determined left ventricular mass in the Framingham Heart Study. *N Engl J Med* 1990;322:1561-1566.

4.   Koren MJ, Devereux RB, Casale PN, et al: Relation of left ventricular mass and geometry to morbidity and mortality in uncomplicated essential hypertension. *Ann Intern Med* 1991;114: 345-352.

5.   Liao Y, Cooper RS, McGee DL, et al: The relative effects of left ventricular hypertrophy, coronary artery disease, and ventricular dysfunction on survival among black adults. *JAMA* 1995;273: 1592-1597.

6.   Beaglehole R, Tyroler HA, Cassel JC, et al: An epidemiologic study of left ventricular hypertrophy in the biracial population of Evans County, Georgia. *J Chronic Dis* 1975;28:549-559.

7.   Rautaharju PM, Park LP, Gottdiener JS, et al: Race- and sex-specific ECG models for left ventricular mass in older populations. Factors influencing overestimation of left ventricular hypertrophy prevalence by ECG criteria in African-Americans. *J Electrocardiol* 2000;33:205-217.

8.   Arnett DK, Strogatz DS, Ephross SA, et al: Greater incidence of electrocardiographic left ventricular hypertrophy in black men than in white men in Evans County, Georgia. *Ethn Dis* 1992;2:10-17.

9.   Xie X, Liu K, Stamler J, et al: Ethnic differences in electrocardiographic left ventricular hypertrophy in young and middle-aged employed American men. *Am J Cardiol* 1994;73:564-567.

10.   Arnett DK, Rautaharju P, Crow R, et al: Black-white differences in electrocardiographic left ventricular mass and its association with blood pressure (the ARIC Study). *Am J Cardiol* 1994;74:247-252.

11.   Rautaharju PM, Zhou S, Calhoun HP: Ethnic differences in ECG amplitudes in North American white, black, and Hispanic men and women. *J Electrocardiol* 1994;27(suppl):20-31.

12.   Vitelli LL, Crow RS, Shafar E, et al: Electrocardiographic findings in a healthy biracial population. *Am J Cardiol* 1998;81: 453-459.

13.   Rautaharju PM, Park LP, Gottdiener JS, et al: Race- and sex-specific ECG models for left ventricular mass in older populations. Factors influencing overestimation of left ventricular hypertrophy prevalence by ECG criteria in African-Americans. *J Electrocardiol* 2000;33:205-217.

14.   Dunn FG, Oigman W, Sungaard-Riise K, et al: Racial differences in cardiac adaptation to essential hypertension determined by echocardiographic indexes. *J Am Coll Cardiol* 1983;5:1348-1351.

15.   Hammond IW, Devereux RB, Alderman MH, et al: The prevalence and correlates of echocardiographic left ventricular hypertrophy among employed patients with uncomplicated hypertension. *J Am Coll Cardiol* 1986;7:639-650.

16.   Liebson PR, Grandits G, Prineas R, et al: Echocardiographic correlates of left ventricular structure among 844 mildly hypertensive men and women in the treatment of mild hypertension study (TOMHS). *Circulation* 1993;87:476-486.

135

17.   Gottdiener JS, Reda DJ, Materson BJ, et al: Importance of obesity, race and age to the cardiac structural and functional effects of hypertension. *J Am Coll Cardiol* 1994;24:1492-98.

18.   Koren MJ, Mensah GA, Blake J, et al: Comparison of left ventricular mass and geometry in black and white patients with essential hypertension. *Am J Hypertens* 1993;6:815-823.

19.   Okin PM, Wright JT, Nieminen MS, et al: Ethnic differences in electrocardiographic criteria for left ventricular hypertrophy: the LIFE Study. *Am J Hypertens* 2002;15:663-671.

20.   Magalski A, Maron BJ, Main ML, et al: Relation of race to electrocardiographic patterns in elite American football players. *J Am Coll Cardiol* 2008;51:2250-2255.

21.   Okin PM, Devereux RB, Lee ET, et al: Electrocardiographic repolarization complexity and abnormality predicts all-cause and cardiovascular mortality in diabetes. The Strong Heart Study. *Diabetes* 2004;53:434-440.

22.   Okin PM, Roman MJ, Lee ET, et al: Combined echocardiographic left ventricular hypertrophy and electrocardiographic ST depression improve prediction of mortality in American Indians. The Strong Heart Study. *Hypertension* 2004;43:769-774.

23.   Jimenez-Corona A, Nelson RG, Sievers ML, et al : Electrocardiographic abnormalities predict deaths from cardiovascular disease and ischemic heart disease in Pima Indians with type 2 diabetes. *Am Heart J* 2006;151:1080-1086

24.   Alkeylani A, Miller DD, Shaw LJ, et al: Influence of race on the prediction of cardiac events with stress technetium-99M Sestamibi tomographic imaging in patients with stable angina pectoris. *Am J Cardiol* 1998;81:293-297.

25.   Hannan EL, Kilburn H, O'Donnell JF, et al: Interracial access to selected cardiac procedures for patients hospitalized with coronary artery disease in New York State. *Med Care* 1991;29:430-441.

26.   McBean AM, Warren JL, Babish JD: Continuing differences in the rates of percutaneous transluminal coronary angioplasty and coronary artery bypass graft surgery between elderly black and white Medicare beneficiaries. *Am Heart J* 1994;127:287-295.

27.   Gillum RF, Gillum BS, Grancis CK: Coronary revascularization and cardiac catheterization in the United States: trends in racial differences. *J Am Coll Cardiol* 1997;29:1557-1562.

28.   Giles WH, Anda RF, Casper ML, et al: Race and sex differences in rates of invasive cardiac procedures in US hospitals. *Arch Intern Med* 1995;155:318-324.

29.   Adams PF, Benson V: Current estimates from the National Health Interview Survey, 1990. National Center for Health Statistics. *Vital Health Stat* 1991;181:1-212.

30.   Chulis GS, Eppig FJ, Hogan MO, et al: Health insurance and the elderly: data from MCBS. *Health Care Financ Rev* 1993;14:163-181.

31.   Chulis GS, Eppig FJ, Poisal JA: Ownership and average premiums for Medicare supplementary insurance policies. *Health Care Financ Rev* 1995;17:255-275.

32.   Hannan EL, van Ryn M, Burke J, et al: Access to coronary artery bypass surgery by race/ethnicity and gender among patients who are appropriate for surgery. *Med Care* 1999;37:68-77.

33.   Lucas FL, DeLorenzo MA, Siewers AE: Temporal trends in the utilization of diagnostic testing and treatments for cardiovascular disease in the United States, 1993-2001. *Circulation* 2006;113:374-379.

34.   Hassapoyannesa CA, Giurgiutiua DV, Eavesa G, et al: Apparent racial disparity in the utilization of invasive testing for risk assessment of cardiac patients undergoing noncardiac surgery. *Cardiovasc Revasc Med* 2006;7:64-69.

35.   Kressin NR, Clark JA, Whittle J, et al: Racial differences in health related beliefs, attitudes, and experience of VA cardiac patients: scale development and application. *Med Care* 2002;40:72-85.

36.   Whittle J, Conigliaro J, Good CB, et al: Do patient preferences contribute to racial differences in cardiovascular procedure use? *J Gen Intern Med* 1997;12:267-273.

37.   Aquilante CL, Humma LM, Yarandi HN, et al: Influence of gender and race on hemodynamic response to dobutamine during dobutamine stress echocardiography. *Am J Cardiol* 2004;94:535-538.

38.   de Simone G, Devereux RB, Koren MJ, et al: Midwall left ventricular mechanics: an independent predictor of cardiovascular risk in arterial hypertension. *Circulation* 1996;93:259-265.

39.   Howard BV, Lee ET, Cowan LD, et al: Coronary heart disease prevalence and its relation to risk factors in American Indians: The Strong Heart Study. *Am J Epidemiol* 1995;142:254-268.

40.   Lee ET, Cowan LD, Welty TK, et al: All-cause mortality and cardiovascular disease mortality in three American Indian popula-

tions, aged 45–74 years, 1984–1988: The Strong Heart Study. *Am J Epidemiol* 1998;147:995-1008.

41. Benjamin EJ, Plehn JF, D'Agostino RB, et al: Mitral annular calcification and the risk of stroke in an elderly cohort. *N Engl J Med* 1992;327:374-379.

42. Kamensky G, Lisy L, Polak E, et al: Mitral annular calcifications and aortic plaques as predictors of increased cardiovascular mortality. *J Cardiol* 2001;37(suppl 1):21- 26.

43. Tenenbaum A, Fisman EZ, Shemesh J, et al: Gender paradox in cardiac calcium deposits in middle-aged and elderly patients: mitral annular and coronary calcifications interrelationship. *Maturitas* 2000;36:35-42.

44. Aronow WS: Mitral annular calcification: significant and worth acting upon. *Geriatrics* 1991;46:73-86.

45. Fox CS, Vasan RS, Parise H, et al: Mitral annular calcification predicts cardiovascular morbidity and mortality: The Framingham Heart Study. *Circulation* 2003;107:1492-1496.

46. Roberts WC: The senile cardiac calcification syndrome. *Am J Cardiol* 1986;58:572-574.

47. Adler Y, Herz I, Vaturi M, et al: Mitral annular calcium detected by transthoracic echocardiography is a marker for high prevalence and severity of coronary artery disease in patients undergoing coronary angiography. *Am J Cardiol* 1998;82:1183-1186.

48. Petty GW, Khandheria BK, Whisnant JP, et al: Predictors of cerebrovascular events and death among patients with valvular heart disease: a population-based study. *Stroke* 2003;31:2628-2635.

49. D'Cruz IA, Cohen HC, Prabhu R, et al: Clinical manifestations of mitral annulus calcification with emphasis on its echocardiographic features. *Am Heart J* 1977;94:367-377.

50. Mellino M, Salcedo EE, Lever HM, et al: Echocardiographic-quantified severity of mitral annular calcification: prognostic correlation to related hemodynamic, valvular, rhythm, and conduction abnormalities. *Am Heart J* 1982;103:222-225.

51. Pomerance A: Pathology of the heart with and without cardiac failure in the aged. *Br Heart J* 1965;27:697-710.

52. Willens HJ, Chirinos JA, Hennekens CH: Prevalence and clinical correlates of mitral annulus calcification in Hispanics and non-Hispanic whites. *J Am Soc Echocardiogr* 2007;20:191-196.

53. Bild DE, Detrano R, Peterson D, et al: Ethnic differences in coronary calcification: the Multi-Ethnic Study of Atherosclerosis (MESA). *Circulation* 2005;111:1313.

54. McClelland RL, Chung H, Detrano R, et al: Distribution of coronary artery calcium by race, gender, and age: results from the Multi-Ethnic Study of Atherosclerosis (MESA). *Circulation* 2006;113:30.

55. Diez Roux AV, Detrano R, Jackson S, et al: Acculturation and socioeconomic position as predictors of coronary calcification in a multiethnic sample. *Circulation* 2005;112:1557.

56. Budoff MJ, Nasir K, Maoa S: Ethnic differences of the presence and severity of coronary atherosclerosis *Atherosclerosis* 2006;187:343-350.

57. Fair JM, Kiazand A, Varady A, et al: Ethnic differences in coronary artery calcium in a healthy cohort aged 60 to 69 years. *Am J Cardiol* 2007;100:981-985.

58. Chu K, Swor R, Jackson R, et al: Race and survival after out-of hospital cardiac arrest in a suburban community. *Ann Emerg Med* 1998;31(4):472-482.

59. Becker LB, Han BH, Meyer PM, et al: Racial differences in the incidence of cardiac arrest and subsequent survival. The CPR Chicago Project. *N Engl J Med* 1993;329(9):600-606.

60. Brookoff D, Kellerman AL, Hackman BB, et al: Do blacks get bystander cardiopulmonary resuscitation as often as whites? *Ann Emerg Med* 1994;24(6):1147-1150.

61. Vadeboncoeur TF, Richman PB, Darkohd M, et al: Bystander cardiopulmonary resuscitation for out-of-hospital cardiac arrest in the Hispanic vs the non-Hispanic populations. *Am J Emerg Med* 2008;26:655-660.

62. Summers RL, Cooper GJ, Carlton FB, et al: Prevalence of atypical chest pain descriptions in a population from the southern United States. *Am J Med Sci* 1999;318:142-145.

63. Bell PD, Hudson S: Equity in the diagnosis of chest pain: race and gender. *Am J Health Behav* 2001;25(1):60-71.

64. Ghali JK, Cooper RS, Kowatly I, et al: Delay between onset of chest pain and arrival to the coronary care unit among minority and disadvantaged patients. *J Natl Med Assoc* 1993;85:180-184.

65. Clark LT, Bellam SV, Shah AH, et al: Analysis of prehospital delay among inner-city patients with symptoms of myocardial infarction:

implications for the therapeutic intervention. *J Natl Med Assoc* 1992;84:931-937.

66.   Cooper RS, Simmons B, Castaner A, et al: Survival rates and prehospital delay during myocardial infarction among black persons. *Am J Cardiol* 1986;57:208-211.

67.   Crawford SL, McGraw SA, Smith KW, et al: Do blacks and whites differ in their use of health care for symptoms of coronary heart disease? *Am J Public Health* 1994;84:957-964.

68.   Johnson PA, Lee TH, Cook EF, et al: Effect of race on the presentation and management of patients with acute chest pain. *Ann Intern Med* 1993;118:593-601.

69.   Taylor HA Jr, Canto JG, Sanderson B, et al: Management and outcomes for black patients with acute myocardial infarction in the reperfusion era. *Am J Cardiol* 1998;82:1019-1023.

70.   Raczynski JM, Taylor H, Cutter G, et al: Diagnoses, symptoms, and attribution of symptoms among black and white inpatients admitted for coronary heart disease. *Am J Public Health* 1994;84: 951-956.

71.   Venkat A, Hoekstra J, Lindsell C, et al: The impact of race on the acute management of chest pain. *Acad Emerg Med* 2003;10: 1199-1208.

72.   Nakamura Y, Moss AJ, Brown MW, et al: Ethnicity and long-term outcome after an acute coronary event. Multicenter Myocardial Ischemia Research Group. *Am Heart J* 1999;138:500-506.

73.   Asher CR, Topol EJ, Moliterno DJ: Insights into the pathophysiology of atherosclerosis prognosis of black Americans who have acute coronary syndromes. *Am Heart J* 1999;138:1073-1081.

74.   Ambrose JA, Fuster V: The risk of coronary occlusion is not proportional to the prior severity of coronary stenosis. *Heart* 1998;79:3-4.

75.   Liao Y, Cooper RS, Cao G, et al: Mortality from coronary heart disease and cardiovascular disease among adult U.S. Hispanics: findings from the National Health Interview Survey (1986 to 1994). *J Am Coll Cardiol* 1997;30(5):1200-1205.

76.   Goff DC, Ramsey DJ, Labarthe DR, et al: Greater case-fatality after myocardial infarction among Mexican Americans and women than among non-Hispanic whites and men: the Corpus Christi Heart Project. *Am J Epidemiol* 1994;139:474-483.

77. Rowland ML, Forthofer RN: Investigation of nonresponse bias: Hispanic Health and Nutrition Examination Survey (National Center for Health Statistics). *Vital Health Stat* 1993;119:1-75.

78. National Center for Health Statistics: Public use data file documentation. National Health Interview Survey Multiple Cause of Death, 1986–1994 survey years: 1-40.

79. Herrera CR, Stern MP, Goff D, et al: Mortality among Hispanics [letter]. *JAMA* 1994;271:1237.

80. Reyes B: Dynamics of immigration: return migration to Western Mexico. San Francisco (CA): Public Policy Institute of California, 1997:1-98.

81. Garg M, Vacek JL, Hallas D: Coronary angioplasty in black and white patients: demographic characteristics and outcomes. *South Med J* 2000;93:1187-1191.

82. Scott NA, Kelsey SF, Detre K, et al: Percutaneous transluminal coronary angioplasty in African-American patients (the National Heart, Lung, and Blood Institute 1985 to 1986 Percutaneous Transluminal Coronary Angioplasty Registry). *Am J Cardiol* 1994;73:1141-1146.

83. Iqbal U, Pinnow EE, Lindsay J: Comparison of six-month outcomes after percutaneous coronary intervention for whites versus African-Americans. *Am J Cardiol* 2001;88:304-305.

84. Douglas JS, King SB, Roubin GS: Technique of percutaneous transluminal angioplasty of the coronary, renal, mesenteric and peripheral arteries. In: JW Hurst, RC Schlant, CE Rackley, et al (eds), *The Heart,* 7th ed. New York, Mc Graw-Hill, 1990, pp 2131-2156.

85. Maynard C, Wright SM, Every NR, et al: Racial differences in outcomes of veterans undergoing percutaneous coronary interventions. *Am Heart J* 2001;142:309-313.

86. Leborgne L, Cheneau E, Wolfram R, et al: Comparison of baseline characteristics and one-year outcomes between African-Americans and Caucasians undergoing percutaneous coronary intervention. *Am J Cardiol* 2004;93(4):389-393.

87. Iqbal U, Pinnow EE, Lindsay J: Comparison of six-month outcomes after percutaneous coronary intervention for whites versus African-Americans. *Am J Cardiol* 2001;88:304-305.

88. Marks DS, Mensah GA, Kennard ED, et al: Race, baseline characteristics, and clinical outcomes after coronary intervention:

141

The new approaches in coronary interventions (NACI) registry. *Am Heart J* 2000;140:162-169.

89. Slater J, Selzer F, Dorbala S, et al: Ethnic differences in the presentation, treatment strategy, and outcomes of percutaneous coronary intervention (a report from the National Heart, Lung, and Blood Institute Dynamic Registry). *Am J Cardiol* 2003;92:773-778.

90. Pradhan J, Schreiber TL, Niraj A, et al: Comparison of five-year outcome in African Americans versus Caucasians following percutaneous coronary intervention. *Catheter Cardiovasc Intervent* 2008;72:36-44.

91. Echols MR, Mahaffey KW, Banerjee A, et al: Racial differences among high-risk patients presenting with non–ST-segment elevation acute coronary syndromes (results from the SYNERGY trial). *Am J Cardiol* 2007;99:315-321.

92. Scirica BM, Moliterno DJ, Every NR, et al: Racial differences in the management of unstable angina: results from the multicenter GUARANTEE registry *Am Heart J* 1999;138:1065-1072.

93. Hutchinson RG, Watson RL, Davis CE, et al: Racial differences in risk factors for atherosclerosis. The ARIC Study. Atherosclerosis Risk in Communities. *Angiology* 1997;48: 279-290.

94. Maynard C, Fisher LD, Passamani ER, et al: Blacks in the Coronary Artery Surgery Study: risk factors and coronary artery disease. *Circulation* 1986;74:64-71.

95. Maynard C, Wright SM, Every NR, et al: Racial differences in outcomes of veterans undergoing percutaneous coronary interventions. *Am Heart J* 2001;142:309-313.

96. Peterson ED, Shaw LK, DeLong ER, et al: Racial variation in the use of coronary-revascularization procedures. Are the differences real? Do they matter? *N Engl J Med* 1997;336:480-486.

97. Carugo S, Giannattasio C, Calchera I, et al: Progression of functional and structural cardiac alterations in young normotensive uncomplicated patients with type 1 diabetes mellitus. *J Hypertens* 2001;19:1675-1680.

98. Factor SM, Borczuk A, Charron MJ, et al: Myocardial alterations in diabetes and hypertension. *Diabetes Res Clin Pract* 1996;31 (suppl):S133-142.

99. Jacobi JA, Parikh SV, McGuire DK, et al: Racial disparity in clinical outcomes following primary percutaneous coronary

intervention for ST elevation myocardial infarction: Influence of process of care. *J Interven Cardiol* 2007;20:182-187.

100. Inagami S, Borrell LN, Wong MD, et al: The New York Academy of Medicine residential segregation and Latino, black and white mortality in New York City Journal of Urban Health: Bulletin of the New York Academy of Medicine. 2006;83(3).

101. Barnhart JM, Fang J, Alderman MH: Differential use of coronary revascularization and hospital mortality following acute myocardial infarction. *Arch Intern Med* 2003;163(4):461-466.

102. AHA Updated statistics, 2008.

103. Vaccarino V, Rathore SS, Wenger NK, et al: Sex and racial differences in the management of acute myocardial infarction, 1994 through 2002. *N Engl J Med* 2005;353:671-682.

104. Cromwell J, McCall NT, Burton J, et al: Race/ethnic disparities in utilization of lifesaving technologies by Medicare ischemic heart disease beneficiaries. *Med Care* 2005;43:330-337.

105. Bridges CR, Edwards FH, Peterson ED, et al: The effect of race on coronary bypass operative mortality. *J Am Coll Cardiol* 2000;36:1870-1976.

106. Brooks MM, Jones RH, Bach RG, et al: Predictors of mortality and mortality from cardiac causes in the bypass angioplasty revascularization investigation (BARI) randomized trial and registry. *Circulation* 2000;101:2682-2689.

107. Yeo KK, Zhongmin L, Amsterdam E: Clinical characteristics and 30-day mortality among Caucasians, Hispanics, Asians, and African-Americans in the 2003 California Coronary Artery Bypass Graft Surgery Outcomes reporting program. *Am J Cardiol* 2007;100:59-63.

108. Correa-de-Araujo R, Stevens B, Moy E, et al: Gender differences across racial and ethnic groups in the quality of care for acute myocardial infarction and heart failure associated with comorbidities. *Women's Health Issues* 2006;16:44-55.

109. Mazar M, Schair B, Aronow WS, et al: Prevalence of use of cardiovascular drugs in 499 patients with suspected coronary artery disease at time of hospitalization for coronary angiography and in 357 Patients with obstructive coronary artery disease documented by coronary angiography. *Am J Ther* 2008;15:458-460.

110. Din-Dzietham R, Couper D, Evans G, et al: Arterial stiffness is greater in African Americans than in whites. *Am J Hypertens* 2004; 17:304-313.

111. Chaturvedi N, McKeigue PM, Marmot MG, et al: A comparison of left ventricular abnormalities associated with glucose intolerance in African Caribbeans and Europeans in the UK. *Heart* 2001; 85;643-648.

112. Houghton JL, Philbin EF, Strogatz DS, et al: The presence of African American race predicts improvement in coronary endothelial function after supplementary L-arginine. *J Am Coll Cardiol* 2002;39:1314-1322.

113. Ergul S, Parish DC, Puett D, et al: Racial differences in plasma endothelin-1 concentrations in individuals with essential hypertension. *Hypertension* 1996;28:652-655.

114. Clark LT: Vascular inflammation as a therapeutic target for prevention of cardiovascular disease. *Curr Atheroscler Rep* 2002;4: 77-81.

115. Albert MA, Torres J, Glynn RJ, et al: Perspective on selected issues in cardiovascular disease research with a focus on black Americans. *Circulation* 2004;110:e7-12.

Chapter 6

Stroke

By Philip R. Liebson, MD

Stroke is a sudden, devastating event that—if it does not kill the victim immediately—leaves him or her with various degrees of disability that affect physical and psychological well-being. It is the third most common cause of death in the United States. Unlike a myocardial infarction, in which the general functioning of ambulation, speech, and thought processes is left intact, stroke can cause permanent damage that produces physical and psychological dependence on caregivers, leads to a sense of isolation unlike most other cardiovascular events, and puts a powerful strain on a family's economic resources. Additionally, there is evidence that the risk for stroke and interventions for stroke victims in special populations may vary. Blacks, Hispanics, American Indians, Alaska Natives, and Asians have a higher mortality at younger ages than do whites.[1] In 2005, the prevalence of stroke among Native Americans (6.0%), multiracial persons (4.6%), and blacks (4.0%) was higher than that for whites (2.3%), with Asians and Hispanics having a similar prevalence as whites. Educational status is also associated with stroke, ranging from 1.8% in college graduates to 4.4% in those with less than 12 years of education.

Stroke has a particularly excessive burden in blacks, especially in the Southeastern US, and in those who are relatively young (35-64 years of age).[2] Of stroke deaths in

2002, 12% occurred in persons under 65 years of age and the proportion of stroke deaths in this younger age group was higher among blacks, Native Americans, and Asians compared with whites.[2] This amounted to 3,400 excess stroke rates in blacks in this younger population compared with whites. Although mortality rates have decreased in both blacks and whites, there remains an unchanging magnitude of the excessive rates in blacks compared with whites.[3]

Although the mortality from stroke in the US population has decreased ever since records were first kept early in the 20th century,[4] the vast increase in population and the increase in average lifespan have led to many more cases. Trends in the age-, race-, and sex-adjusted prevalence of stroke between 1971 and 1994 from the National Health and Nutrition Examination Surveys (NHANES I to NHANES III) demonstrated an increase from 1.4% to 1.9%, an average increase of 7.5%.[4] In terms of actual numbers, noninstitutionalized stroke survivors increased by 60% during this period, from 1.5 million to 2.4 million. As for racial differences, 5-year mean change in stroke prevalence in noninstitutionalized survivors of stroke increased by 28% in black women and 12% in white men, but decreased by 3% in black men and by 3% in white women. However, in terms of estimated noninstitutional stroke survivors, 5-year changes in numbers of survivors increased in all groups, from an increase of 18,000 in black males to 159,000 in white males. These differences, of course, were accounted for by the 10-fold larger population of whites than blacks.

An intriguing finding in terms of possible environmental implications is that the stroke death rate is particularly high in the Southeastern US.[5] Geographic differences in stroke prevalence may relate to cultural differences in diet and exercise, lack of economic opportunity, and regional differences in health care and preventive services. Both environmental risk factors and new evidence for genetic determinants leading to risk for stroke in special populations must be considered in evaluation of preventive interventions.

Incidence, Prevalence, and Risk for Stroke in Blacks

The 'stroke belt' was identified in 1965 in the southeastern US as a region that had a 50% higher stroke mortality rate.[6] This higher rate was evaluated by a 2003 Behavioral Risk Factor Surveillance System (BRFSS) survey.[2] A comparison was made among Southeastern and non-Southeastern states. A total of 95,598 persons responded, including substantial numbers of blacks and whites. The highest age-adjusted prevalence of stroke was found in southeastern blacks (3.4%), followed by non-southeastern blacks (2.8%), southeastern whites (2.5%), and non-southeastern whites (1.8%). Characteristics of southeastern blacks that might explain their increased stroke prevalence compared to whites include lower education levels and higher prevalence of diabetes and high blood pressure. Health insurance coverage among blacks is also lower in the region compared to whites and to those in non-southeastern states. Other considerations in the southeastern states that have been advanced for regional variations include lower intakes of animal protein, potassium, and calcium, and higher intakes of sodium and complex carbohydrates.

More recent evaluations of black populations in southern states indicate a black-to-white stroke mortality ratio that is 6% to 21% higher in these states than in non-southern states, and even in southern states not part of the stroke belt (Virginia, Florida, and the lower Mississippi region).[6]

The higher stroke prevalence rate in blacks versus whites has been confirmed in a number of incidence studies. In a 1993-1994 population-based study in the Greater Cincinnati/Northern Kentucky region, fairly representative of demographic and socioeconomic characteristics, stroke incidence in blacks was higher at any age with the greatest risk, 2-fold to 5-fold, in young and middle-aged blacks compared to whites.[7] In terms of the type of stroke (ischemic, intracerebral hemorrhage, and subarachnoid hemorrhage), the race-specific incidence rates were higher for all categories in blacks, with a hazard ratio of 1.8 to 2.0 compared with whites. This racial disparity was accounted for by the higher prevalence of risk factors for stroke in blacks such as hypertension, diabetes, smoking, and alcohol use, as well as decreased access to health care, all of which are similar to risk factors in the southern stroke belt.

In terms of stroke locations, a relative excess of small vessel intracranial disease was found in black patients with stroke compared with an excess of extracranial atherosclerosis and cardioembolic stroke in whites, independent of conventional risk factors and social class.

Hispanics

Less study has been done on stroke characterization in Hispanics, although they are now considered the largest minority population in the US. Mexican Americans constitute by far the largest subgroup of Hispanic Americans and as such have been exclusively evaluated as representative of Hispanic populations in the NHANES surveys.

In 1990, cerebrovascular disease (CVD) was the fourth leading cause of deaths in Hispanics in the US. At that time, stroke deaths were similar between middle-aged (45-64 years of age) Hispanics and non-Hispanic whites but substantially lower in Hispanics at ages 65 and older.[8] At the time, Hispanics had lower levels of hypertension and hypercholesterolemia than non-Hispanic whites but higher levels of diabetes, smoking, and overweight.

More recently, the stroke incidence among Mexican Americans and non-Hispanic whites was evaluated in a Texas county from January 2000 to December 2002 as part of the Brain Attack Surveillance in Corpus Christi Project (BASIC).[9] Mexican Americans had a 24% higher cumulative incidence of strokes than non-Hispanic whites (168/10,000 vs 136/10,000). This included a higher incidence of both ischemic and intracerebral stroke. Subarachnoid hemorrhage was also more common but was of borderline statistical significance.

In the BASIC study, subarachnoid hemorrhage dispro-portionately affected Mexican Americans and women, although no ethnic difference was found in in-hospital mortality or discharge disability.[10] Aside from increased vascular malformations in Hispanics, other possible reasons include increased prevalence of hypertension, heavy alcohol consumption, and cigarette smoking in Hispanics. For gender differences, possible explanations have included differences in hypertension, smoking, and estrogen effects in women.

In comparative studies of intracerebral hemorrhages in Mexican Americans and non-Hispanic whites in the BASIC project, Mexican Americans were more likely to have smaller, nonlobar hemorrhages.[11] Hispanics had a higher prevalence of diabetes and a lower prevalence of coronary artery disease. The higher, characteristic nonlobar stroke incidence in Mexican Americans may relate to a possible increased risk for this pathology in diabetics.

Inter- and Intraracial Variations

The relative incidence of strokes among blacks, Hispanics, and whites has been evaluated in the Northern Manhattan Study (NOMAS).[12] An evaluation of ischemic stroke between 1993-1997 in that part of New York City demonstrated increased incidences of stroke subtypes in both blacks and Hispanics compared with non-Hispanic whites. This difference was as high as an annual age-adjusted intracranial atherosclerotic stroke risk ratio of 5:1 in both blacks and Hispanics compared to non-Hispanic whites, but also included increased risk ratios in both minority groups for extracranial atherosclerotic stroke, lacunar stroke, and cardioembolic stroke. Another salient feature was the younger age of the minority groups at the time of first stroke compared with whites (66 years for Hispanics, 71 years for blacks, 77 years for whites). As reflected in other analyses, the prevalence of stroke risk factors in both minority ethnic groups—such as hypertension, hypercholesterolemia, and smoking—was much higher than in whites. The only stroke subcategory in which whites had a greater risk was cardioembolic stroke, reflecting the greater prevalence of atrial fibrillation in whites than among blacks and Hispanics.

In a further evaluation of risk factors in the Northern Manhattan Study, variations in risk of stroke were found in the various ethnic groups. Although hypertension was an independent risk factor for all three ethnic groups, the greater prevalence of hypertension in blacks and Hispanics led to a higher etiologic fraction of risk or attributable risk (37% and 31%, respectively) than in whites (25%).[13] Greater prevalence of diabetes led to increased risk in blacks (21%) and Caribbean Hispanics (20%), compared with whites (11%) adjusted for age, sex, and other risk factors. Coronary artery disease and atrial fibrillation, on the other hand, provided a larger proportion of risk for whites (16% and 20%, respectively) than the other two groups (6% or lower for risk in both conditions for blacks and Hispanics).

Native Americans

Relatively few studies have evaluated stroke in Native Americans. This ethnic population has a relatively high rate of tobacco abuse, diabetes, hypertension, and elevated cholesterol levels.[14] The rates of stroke are higher for Native Americans than for US whites. Cerebrovascular disease is the sixth leading cause of death in this population, with adjusted rates of 29.6/100,000 versus 24.0 for whites.[15] Although the risk factors for CVD are higher in Native Americans than in whites, national vital event data suggest a lower mortality for this ethnic/racial group than the general US population. The concern about this finding is the possibility of racial misclassification. Focused epidemiologic studies on Native American populations, such as the Strong Heart Study, suggest that CVD incidence and mortality rates in Native Americans are as bad as or worse than that of general US population.[15] A study by the National Center for Health Statistics found an underestimation of death rates of 21% for Native Americans, 11% for Asians, and 2% for Hispanics, but an overestimation by 5% for blacks and 1% for whites.[16]

There is evidence from an evaluation of Montana Native Americans and whites between 1991-2000 that stroke mortality declined significantly in whites during that period (from 64 to 60/100,000) but increased slightly in Native Americans (80 to 81/100,000).[17]

In general, the prevalence of CVD risk factors among US ethnic groups is second highest among Native Americans (47%), after blacks (49%).[18] In the entire US, stroke mortality in Native Americans increased from 41 to 45/100,000 from 1990 to 2000.[17] In the Montana study, stroke mortality in Native Americans was 2-fold higher than for all other races combined on a national level, and comparable to the national stroke mortality rate for US blacks. One must consider the heterogeneity of Native American tribes in evaluating these statistics, and further studies must be conducted on possible disparities in stroke incidence among various Native American populations.

The recent report from the Strong Heart Study provides an update of incidence and risk factors for stroke in the Native American population.[19] This is the largest longitudinal, population-based study of CVD and its risk factors in a diverse group of Native Americans. The study covered the period from 1989-1992, when baseline examinations were accomplished, through December 2004. Nonhemorrhagic ischemic infarction occurred in 86% of stroke victims, hemorrhagic stroke in the rest. The incidence rate and case fatality rate were found to be higher than in US white and black populations of the same age range. Hypertension, diabetes, and smoking were strongly associated with stroke, as was to be expected.

Asians had similar risks than those of whites. Infants (<1-year old) had the highest annual stroke rates for ischemic stroke and intracerebral hemorrhage of any age group. Boys were at higher risk of all types of strokes than were girls. Excess stroke risk persisted for blacks after eliminating sickle cell disease, and persisted for boys after eliminating trauma. Despite these differences, case fatality rates were similar in all racial groups, but in gender comparisons, boys had a higher case fatality rate than girls.

A recent epidemiologic report from the International Pediatric Stroke Study provides preliminary information on ischemic stroke in children (from neonates to 19 years of age).[20] The information is derived from a registry that began in 2003 and included data through July 2007. Among 1,187 children with confirmed stroke, male predominance was seen at all ages (61% for neonates, 59% for later childhood). This was found with all ischemic stroke subtypes, and although slightly increased rates in males were associated with trauma, the difference persisted when trauma was taken into account. The male predominance has been attributed to increased vasculitis (in male children), neuroprotective effects of estrogen, and increased risk of trauma.[20] However, these attributes are tenuous and it is possible that X-linked and endocrine factors not yet evaluated might explain these gender differences.

Genetics

A family history of stroke is a risk factor for CVD. This is especially so in probands and relatives <70 years of age.[21] There is evidence that the heritability of ischemic versus hemorrhagic stroke may be different. Ischemic stroke is thought to have a polygenic basis. Familial aggregation of stroke may be due to intermediate phenotypes, including diabetes and hypertension, also aggregating in families. It appears that there is some racial variation in familial aggregation. For example, the BASIC project found that Mexican Americans with stroke were twice as likely to have a sibling with stroke as non-Hispanic whites.[22]

Considerable interest has arisen about the possible heritability differences of stroke in different racial groups and in women. Polymorphisms that may affect warfarin activity have already been referred to. Associations of various polymorphisms influencing risk for stroke have been investigated in blacks, Hispanics, and Asians. The greatest harvests are reaped in studying candidate genes from younger patients with stroke. Unfortunately, most of the studies have been limited in power because of small sample sizes.

An example of a genetic marker for strokes in blacks is the intron 4c allele of the endothelial nitric oxide (NOS3) gene.[23] Intron 4c is overrepresented in stroke patients and appears to be most strongly associated with large artery ischemic stroke in black Americans.

Another candidate gene as a risk marker for incident stroke is the cyclooxygenase-2 (COX-2) G-765C variant.[24] Inflammation may be mediated by the COX enzyme. The genotype was found to be a significant predictor of incident stroke in black Americans but not whites in a population in the Atherosclerosis Risk in Communities (ARIC) study.

Phosphodiesterase 4D polymorphisms have been studied in black and white women. A single nucleotide polymorphism (SNP res918592) was significantly associated with stroke in blacks and whites across multiple stroke subtypes.[25] The interesting finding in this association was that it was confined exclusively to current smokers. It is possible that smoking can modify gene expression in endothelial cells.

Studies have also focused on genetic susceptibilities to stroke in Asians, especially those of Chinese and Japanese ancestry. A study in the United Kingdom of ischemic stroke among 32,500 persons of non-European descent, mainly Chinese, Japanese, and Korean individuals, with a meta-analysis of eight candidate genes, suggested that genetic associations studied for ischemic stroke in these racial groups were similar to those of European descent.[26]

Three genes associated with ischemic stroke included the ACE insertion/deletion polymorphism, the C677T variant of methylenetetrahydrofolate reductase, and the apolipoprotein E gene, variably significantly associated with stroke in the three Asian groups, as well as in those of European descent. As with other studies of this type, the concern about genetic associations for stroke relates to the limited number of gene variants evaluated, the small number of individuals in each study, and the possibility of publication bias.

Parallel with the UK meta-analysis, similar susceptibility loci for intracranial aneurysm, a risk factor for hemorrhagic stroke, was found when comparing Japanese individuals with Finnish and Dutch cohorts.[27] Common SNPs on three chromosomes showed a significant association with intracranial aneurysms in all three groups. Presumably, the associated SNPs act via pathways required for formation and maintenance of endothelial cells.

The heritability of carotid distensibility, a risk factor for atherosclerosis and stroke, was evaluated in a high-risk Caribbean Hispanic population in the NOMAS study.[28] After age and sex adjustment, heritability was 25% for carotid vascular strain characteristics, 17% for distensibility, 20% for stiffness, and 20% for elastic modulus. Although there was a correlation between distensibility and carotid intimal-medial thickness (IMT), the correlation was considerably reduced with adjustment for age and sex. The results suggest that although there is a substantial heritability in carotid distensibility, the age and sex variability outweighs its impact on carotid IMT, the latter relating more substantially to the possibility of future stroke. The Strong Heart Study also found a substantial heritability for carotid stiffness in Native Americans.[29]

Prognosis

The prognosis of stroke in racial groups varies considerably, just as its epidemiology and prevalence. Much of the variation is due to health disparities related not only to ethnicity, but also to regional variations. Recent evidence bolsters the evidence for a greater burden of disease in stroke, greater mortality, and greater severity of strokes in blacks.[30] Less conclusive is evidence for differences in acute and postacute care as well as disparities among other ethnic groups.

Regarding the stroke belt in southeastern US, higher stroke mortality occurs in both blacks and whites, although there is some racial variation in risk factors.[31] For example, regional cigarette smoking by whites is highest in the southeastern region, but not in blacks.[31] As discussed previously, other explanations for the high stroke rate in the southeastern US include a lower potassium and calcium diet (especially pronounced among blacks) and lower animal protein and higher grain-derived complex carbohydrate diets with increased sodium intake, similar to diets in Japan with its high stroke mortality.

In regard to stroke mortality, US age-adjusted death rates from 1999 were 35% higher in blacks than in non-Hispanic whites. In data from the late 1990s, mortality rates for intracerebral hemorrhage were 1.7 times higher in blacks and 1.5 times higher in Asian/Pacific Islanders than in whites.[30] Although stroke deaths have declined over the past few decades, rates of decline in black men are lower.

Stroke mortality was the third leading cause of death in black men and the sixth in black women in the US in 1996.[32] Age-adjusted death rates for stroke per 100,000 were 50.9 for black men, 39.2 for black women, 22.9 for white women, and 26.3 for white men. Stroke death rates for blacks in the 1990s were similar to rates in Japan, but lower than those in Eastern Europe. Stroke mortality rates for blacks in Africa and the Caribbean region are also relatively high but there are concerns about possible death certification inaccuracies and demographic analysis in these regions. Recently, there has been a slowdown in the decline of US stroke mortality in both blacks and whites (Figure 6-1).

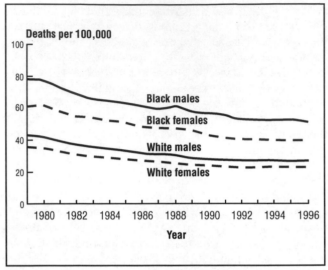

Figure 6-1: National Center for Health Statistics. Age-adjusted stroke mortality rates in the United States, 1979-1996. Since the early 1980s, a marked slowdown has occurred in the decline in US stroke mortality in black and white Americans.

Conclusions

The variations of stroke risk, incidence, prevalence, and prognosis in minority groups compared with whites, as well as gender and age differences, have been attributed to differences in heritable and environmental factors, not the least important being lifestyle choices. These considerations are important in dealing with interventions to modify stroke risk.

Primary prevention of stroke is clearly the best approach to intervention and requires flexibility for different racial groups. For example, church-based programs have been successful in screening for hypertension in black individuals. A pilot project to assess the need for and feasibility of a church-based stroke risk reduction intervention was recently reported.[33] Of a total of 150 Mexican Americans (63%) and non-Hispanic whites evaluated after several masses over one weekend, 84% expressed interest in a long-term church-based health education project. Blood pressure was elevated in 25% of individuals without known hypertension, and even in those with established hypertension, 64% had elevated blood pressures, indicating inadequate control. Mexican Americans were more likely to be overweight and have diabetes than non-Hispanic whites. As with other church-based health programs, female participation was greater than that of men.

Stroke burden in the US can be reduced by a combination of interventions, including the primary prevention and control of risk factors, catered to the cultural characteristics of individual racial/ethnic groups; public education about the signs and symptoms of stroke; the need for emergency response and rapid transport to a stroke center; and effective rehabilitation and secondary prevention in stroke victims.[34]

The major efforts involve control of smoking, hypertension, diabetes, and lipid abnormalities. In this way, it is possible that the proposed US goal for health promotion and disease prevention for 2010, in terms of stroke deaths, will lead to no more than 51 per 100,000 population for each population group.[32]

References

1.   Centers for Disease Control and Prevention (CDC): Prevalence of stroke—United States 2005. *MMWR* 2007;56:469-474.

2.   Centers for Disease Control and Prevention (CDC): Regional and racial differences in prevalence of stroke—23 states and District of Columbia, 2003. *MMWR* 2005;54:481-484.

3.   Howard G, Howard VJ: Ethnic disparities in stroke: the scope of the problem. *Ethnic Dis* 2001;11:761-768

4.   Muntner P, Garrett E, Klag MJ, et al: Trends in stroke prevalence between 1973 and 1991 in the US population 25 to 74 years of age. *Stroke* 2002;33:1209-1213.

5.   Lanska DJ, Kuller LH: The geography of stroke mortality in the United States and the concept of a stroke belt. *Stroke* 1995;26:1145-1149.

6.   Howard G, Labarthe DR, Hu J, et al: Regional differences in African Americans' high risk for stroke: the remarkable burden of stroke for Southern African Americans. *Ann Epidemiol* 2007;17: 689-696.

7.   Kissela B, Schneider A, Kleindorfer D, et al: Stroke in bi-racial population. The excess burden of stroke in blacks. *Stroke* 2004;35:426-431.

8.   Gillum RF: Epidemiology of stroke in Hispanic Americans. *Stroke* 1995;26:1707-1712.

9.   Morgenstern LB, Smith MA, Lisabeth LD, et al: Excess stroke in Mexican Americans compared with non-Hispanic Whites: the Brain Attack Surveillance in Corpus Christi Project. *Am J Epidemiol* 2004;160:376-383.

10.   Eden SV, Meurer WJ, Sánchez BN, et al: Gender and ethnic differences in subarachnoid hemorrhage. *Neurology* 2008;71:731-735.

11.   Zahuranec DB, Brown DL, Lisabeth LD, et al: Differences in intracerebral hemorrhage between Mexican Americans and non-Hispanic whites. *Neurology* 2006;66:30-34.

12.   White H, Boden-Albala B, Wang C, et al: Ischemic stroke subtype incidence among whites, blacks, and Hispanics: the Northern Manhattan Study. *Circulation* 2005;111:1327-1331.

13.   Sacco RL, Boden-Albala B, Abel G, et al: Race-ethnic disparities in the impact of stroke risk factors: the northern Manhattan stroke study. *Stroke* 2001;32:1725-1731.

14.   Galloway JM: Cardiovascular health among American Indians and Alaska Natives: successes, challenges, and potentials. *Am J Prev Med* 2005;29(suppl 5):11-17.

15.   Rhoades DA: Racial misclassification and disparities in cardiovascular disease among American Indians and Alaska natives. *Circulation* 2005;111:1250-1256.

16.   Rosenberg HM, Mauerer JD, Sorlie PD, et al: Quality of death rates by race and Hispanic-origin: a summary of current research, 1999. *Vital Health Stat* 1999;2:1-14.

17.   Harwell TS, Oser CS, Okon NJ, et al: Defining disparities in cardiovascular disease for American Indians: trends in heart disease

and stroke mortality among American Indians and whites in Montana, 1991 to 2000. *Circulation* 2005;112:2263-2267.

18. Centers for Disease Control and Prevention (CDC): Racial/ethnic and socioeconomic disparities in multiple risk factors for heart disease and stroke–United States, 2003. *MMWR* 2003;52:1-13.

19. Zhang Y, Galloway JM, Welty TK, et al: Incidence and risk factors for stroke in American Indians: the Strong Heart Study. *Circulation* 2008;118:1577-1584.

20. Golomb MR, Fullerton HJ, Nowak-Gottl U, deVeber G, for the International Pediatric Stroke Study Group: Male predominance in childhood ischemic stroke. *Stroke* 2009;40:52-57.

21. Flossmann E, Schultz UGR, Rothwell PM: Systematic review of methods and results of studies of the genetic epidemiology of ischemic stroke. *Stroke* 2004;35:212-227.

22. Lisabeth LD, Kardia SLR, Smith MAS, et al: Family history of stroke among Mexican-American and non-Hispanic White patients with stroke and TIA: Implications for the feasibility and design of stroke genetics research. *Neuroepidemiology* 2005;24:96-102.

23. Grewal RP, Dutra AV, Liao YC, et al: The intron 4c allele of the NOS3 gene is associated with ischemic stroke in African Americans. *BMC Med Genet* 2007;8:76.

24. Kohsaka S, Volcik KA, Folsom ZAR, et al: Increased risk of incident stroke associated with the cyclooxygenase 2 (COX-2) G-765C polymorphism in African-Americans; the Atherosclerosis Risk in Communities study. *Atherosclerosis* 2008;196:926-930.

25. Song Q, Cole JW, O'Connell JR, et al: Phosphodiesterase 4D polymorphisms and the risk of cerebral infarction in a biracial population; the Stroke Prevention in Young Women Study. *Hum Mol Genet* 2006;15:2468-2478.

26. Ariyaratam R, Casas JP, Whittaker J, et al: Genetics of ischaemic stroke among persons of non-European descent: A meta-analysis of eight genes involving ≈ 32,500 individuals. *PLoS Medicine* 2007;4:0728-0736.

27. Bilguvar K, Yasuno K, Niemelä M, et al: Susceptibility loci for intracranial aneurysm in European and Japanese populations. *Nat Genet* 2008;40:1472-1477.

28. Juo S-HH, Rundek T, Lin H-F, et al: Heritability of carotid artery distensibility in Hispanics. The Northern Manhattan Family Study. *Stroke* 2005;36:2357-2361.

29.   North KE, MacCluer JW, Devereux RB, et al: Heritability of carotid artery structure and function: the Strong Heart Family Study. *Arterioscler Thromb Vasc Biol* 2002;22:1698-1703.

30.   Stansbury JP, Jia H, Williams LS, et al: Ethnic disparities in stroke: epidemiology, acute care, and postacute outcomes. *Stroke* 2005;36:364-386.

31.   Pickle LW, Mungiole M, Gillum RF: Geographic variation in stroke mortality in blacks and whites in the United States. *Stroke* 1997;28:1639-1647.

32.   Gillum RF: Stroke mortality in blacks. Disturbing trends. *Stroke* 1999;30:1711-1715.

33.   Zahuranec DB, Morgenstern LB, Garcia NM, et al: Stroke health and risk education (SHARE) pilot project. *Stroke* 2008;39:1583-1585.

34.   McGruder HF, Malarcher AM, Antoine TL, et al: Racial and ethnic disparities in cardiovascular risk factors among stroke survivors. United States 1999-2001. *Stroke* 2004;35:1557-1561.

Chapter 7

Heart Failure

By C. Tissa Kappagoda, MD, PhD,
and Ezra A. Amsterdam, MD

Heart failure (HF) is defined as a condition in which the heart is unable to pump sufficient blood to meet the needs of the body.[1] We now recognize that the pathophysiologic basis of HF is systolic dysfunction, diastolic dysfunction, or a combination of these two abnormalities. Systolic HF results from impaired ventricular contractile function, while diastolic HF is caused by reduced ventricular compliance that causes elevated filling pressures at normal ventricular volumes. The signs and symptoms of HF fall into two categories: (1) the consequences of disturbances in the pulmonary circulation, and (2) result of changes in the neuroendocrine systems, such as the renin-angiotensin-aldosterone (RAA) axis, that play essential roles in the regulation of salt and water metabolism and vascular function through their actions on the heart, kidneys, and blood vessels. Heart failure disturbs the balance of Starling forces that regulate fluid fluxes between the microcirculation and the extravascular compartment of the airways and lungs.[2] The precise nature of these changes in Starling forces depends on the ventricle involved. Another potentially complicating factor is that failure of each ventricle may be due to systolic dysfunction, diastolic dysfunction, or both. Often, when the left ventricle is involved, it is difficult to distinguish these two forms of failure clinically, because the resulting signs and symptoms are often qualitatively similar (though different in degree).

The clinical manifestations associated with left ventricular failure include tachypnea, dyspnea (accompanied by an associated sense of distress), fatigue, bronchospasm, and cough.[1] These features are preceded by an increase in the volume of fluid in the extravascular space of the lung. Paroxysmal nocturnal dyspnea is a particular manifestation of left ventricular failure when the extravascular fluid accumulates in the lung at night after the subject assumes a horizontal position during sleep. The most consistent hemodynamic feature of left ventricular failure, regardless of its etiology, is an increase in left atrial pressure, which in turn leads to a disturbance of the Starling forces in a manner that favors an increase in extravascular fluid in the airways and lungs.

In right ventricular failure, the hydrostatic pressure increases in the right atrium and the vena cavae. The hydrostatic pressures in the microcirculation of the lung are not affected to the same extent as in left ventricular failure, and respiratory symptoms are not usually pronounced in patients with right ventricular failure. However, homeostasis of the extravascular fluid volume of the airways and lungs also depends on effective pulmonary lymph drainage. The pumping pressure in the lymphatic vessels close to the external jugular vein is approximately 17 cmH_2O.[3] When this pressure is exceeded in the jugular veins, it is likely that pulmonary lymphatic drainage will be compromised, leading to an increase in the extravascular fluid volume and the appearance of respiratory symptoms.

The second component of the syndrome of HF is the homeostatic mechanisms activated by the reduction in cardiac output (Figure 7-1). The sympathetic nervous system is activated, which manifests itself principally as an increase in vascular tone, heart rate, and contractility to support circulatory function. There is also a concurrent modification of renal function, leading to the retention of

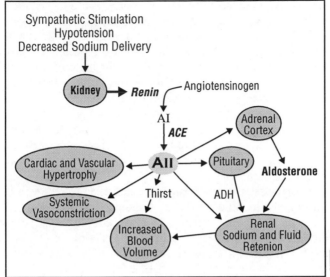

Figure 7-1: The renin-angiotensin-aldosterone system and its relationship to the pathophysiology of heart failure. The primary site of renin storage and release in the body are juxtaglomerular (JG) cells associated with the afferent arteriole of the glomerulus. A reduction in afferent arteriolar pressure causes release of renin from the JG cells, whereas increased pressure inhibits it. β_1-adrenoceptors located on the JG cells also respond to sympathetic nerve stimulation by releasing renin. Specialized cells (macula densa) of distal tubules lie adjacent to the JG cells of the afferent arteriole. The macula densa senses the amount of sodium and chloride ions in the tubular fluid. When NaCl is elevated in the tubular fluid, renin release is inhibited. In contrast, a reduction in tubular NaCl stimulates renin release by the JG cells. Prostaglandins (PGE_2 and PGI_2) stimulate renin release in response to reduced NaCl transport across the macula densa. When afferent arteriole pressure is reduced, glomerular filtration decreases, and this reduces NaCl in the distal tubule. This serves as an important mechanism contributing to the release of renin when there is afferent arteriole hypotension as in heart failure. ACE=angiotensin-converting enzyme, AI=angiotensin I, AII=angiotensin II, ADH=antidiuretic hormone.

163

salt and water in the body. The natural response to the latter is an increase in renal perfusion to restore fluid volume. In HF, this step is aborted due to activation of the RAA system (Figure 7-1). There are three important components to the RAA system: (1) renin, (2) angiotensin, and (3) aldosterone. Renin, a proteolytic enzyme, is released into the circulation primarily by the kidneys. Its release is stimulated by a reduction in the perfusion pressure in the afferent arteriole of the glomerulus, which releases renin from the juxtaglomerular (JG) cells in the arteriole by stimulation of β_1-adrenoceptors. Renin acts upon a circulating substrate, angiotensinogen, which undergoes proteolytic cleavage to form the decapeptide angiotensin I. Vascular endothelium in several tissues, particularly in the lungs, contains angiotensin-converting enzyme (ACE) that cleaves two amino acids to form the octapeptide, angiotensin II (AII). Angiotensin II, in turn, stimulates the release of aldosterone from the adrenal cortex. Angiotensin II also constricts the efferent artery of the glomerulus to maintain glomular filtration pressure. Renin is also released by JG cells in response to a decrease in sodium delivery to the distal tubules of the kidney.

The other component of the system is a group of specialized cells (macula densa) of the renal distal tubules, which lie adjacent to the JG cells of the afferent arteriole. The macula densa senses the amount of sodium and chloride ions in the tubular fluid. When afferent arteriole pressure is reduced, as in HF, glomerular filtration decreases and this reduces sodium chloride (NaCl) in the distal tubule, which serves as an important mechanism contributing to the release of renin when there is afferent arteriole hypotension. When NaCl is elevated in the tubular fluid, renin release is inhibited.

In HF, these potentially beneficial homeostatic mechanisms are distorted in several ways. Angiotensin II: (1) constricts resistance vessels (via AII receptors), thereby increasing systemic vascular resistance (afterload) and arterial pressure, (2) acts on the adrenal cortex to release aldosterone, which in turn acts on the kidneys to increase sodium and fluid retention, (3) stimulates the release of vasopressin (antidiuretic hormone, ADH) from the posterior pituitary, which increases fluid retention by the kidneys, (4) stimulates thirst centers within the brain, (5) facilitates norepinephrine release from sympathetic nerve endings and inhibits norepinephrine re-uptake by nerve endings, thereby enhancing sympathetic adrenergic function, and (6) stimulates cardiac hypertrophy and vascular hypertrophy, now recognized as deleterious remodeling. Taken collectively, these effects increase afterload on the heart and compromise cardiac function further, while simultaneously causing retention of salt and water. These effects provide the rationale for the current approach to management of HF, which is based on reduction of vascular tone, by inhibition of renin-angiotensin and sympathoadrenal systems and, where appropriate, the use of inotropic agents. The RAA pathway is regulated not only by the mechanisms that stimulate renin release, but also by natriuretic peptides (ANP and BNP) released by the heart. These natriuretic peptides act as an important counterregulatory system.

Ischemic cardiomyopathy causes most cases of HF in the United States. Thus, prevention of coronary artery disease (CAD) and myocardial infarction (MI) is an important aspect of reducing the toll of HF. We now know that diastolic HF (HF with normal systolic function) is frequent, accounting for ~30% of cases. However, diastolic dysfunction is also a frequent accompaniment of systolic dysfunction.

Prevalence of HF

The fact sheet on HF produced by the National Institutes of Health (NIH) in 1996 showed that an estimated 4.8 million Americans had congestive HF (CHF). Their five-year mortality was approximately 50%. Each year, there were an estimated 400,000 new cases. The annual number of deaths directly from CHF increased from 10,000 in 1968 to 42,000 in 1993, with another 219,000 related to the condition.[4]

The recent fact sheet from the Centers for Disease Control and Prevention (CDC) (Figure 7-2) highlights the following[5]:

- Approximately 5 million people in the US have HF. About 550,000 new cases are diagnosed each year. More than 287,000 people in the US die each year with HF.
- Hospitalizations for HF have increased substantially, rising from 402,000 in 1979 to 1.1 million in 2004 (National Hospital Discharge Survey).
- HF is the most common reason for hospitalization among people on Medicare. Hospitalizations for HF are higher in black than in white people on Medicare.
- The most common causes of HF are CAD, hypertension, and diabetes. About 7 of 10 people with HF had high blood pressure before being diagnosed. About 22% of men and 46% of women will develop HF within 6 years of having a heart attack.

This rather grim trend has prompted the American Heart Association (AHA) and the American College of Cardiology (ACC) to emphasize the role of prevention in the overall management of HF. They have advocated moving away from the traditional New York Heart Association (NYHA) classification of symptoms to a staging system that emphasizes the evolution of HF (Figure 7-3). Despite numerous clinical trials indicating therapeutic efficacy of various pharmaceutical agents, the overall mortality from HF still remains high (Figure 7-4).[6] To reduce HF mortality, the risk factors leading to the development of HF must be treated effectively, particularly by focusing on ethnic groups that are most at risk.

Heart Failure in African Americans

A recent report from the Atherosclerosis Risk in Communities (ARIC) cohort has provided information about the incidence of HF among African Americans.[6] The ARIC

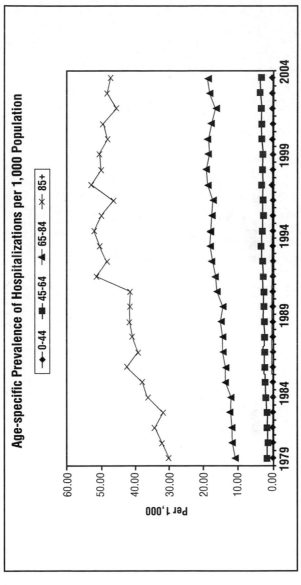

Figure 7-2: Hospitalizations for heart failure in the US. Accessible at: http://www.cdc.gov/dhdsp/library/fs_heart_failure.htm

167

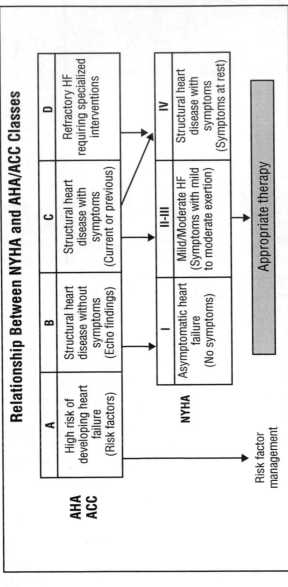

Figure 7-3: The grading of heart failure: reconciling the New York Heart Association Classification with the American Heart Association/American College of Cardiology stages.

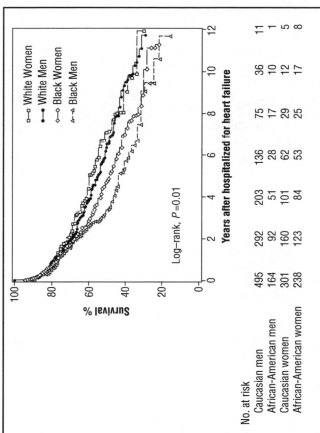

Figure 7-4: Kaplan-Meier survival curves after incident heart failure hospitalization (n=1,206, not including the 76 incident heart failure deaths), stratified by race and gender group, ARIC, 1987 to 2002.[6] Note the high 5-year mortality in all groups.

was a population-based study from four US communities (1987-2002). People with pre-existing HF (n=750) were identified by self-report and were excluded from this analysis. Incident cases of HF were defined in accordance with the International Classification of Diseases codes for HF (428.0-428.9, I50) from a hospitalization or death certificate. There were 1,282 incident HF cases over 198,417 person-years. Age-adjusted incidence rates for HF were greater for African Americans than for Caucasians, but adjustment for confounders attenuated the difference. Thirty-day, 1-year, and 5-year case fatalities following hospitalization for HF were 10.4%, 22%, and 42.3%, respectively. African Americans had a greater 5-year case fatality compared with Caucasians ($P < 0.05$). Overall incidence rates in African-American women were closer to those of men than of Caucasian women. The greater incidence of HF in African Americans than in Caucasians was largely explained by the higher prevalence of atherosclerotic risk factors in African Americans and the greater vulnerability of African Americans to these risk factors, especially hypertension (see Chapter 3).

This increased incidence of HF among African Americans was also reported in elderly individuals in the Aging, Health and Body Composition study that was undertaken in highly functional individuals between 70 and 79 years of age.[7] Over a mean 5.7 years of observation, 7.7% of blacks (87 of 1,124) and 6.7% of whites (113 of 1,676) developed HF, with a higher incidence for blacks than for whites (14.0 events per 1,000 person-years vs 11.6 per 1,000 person-years; $P < 0.001$). Decreased kidney function was associated with the risk of HF in the entire cohort. Individuals with the highest quintile of each marker of kidney function were at twice the risk of HF (compared with those in the lowest quintile), even after adjusting for demographic factors, comorbid conditions, and medications.

The higher prevalence of HF associated with hypertension in African Americans may be related to more impaired diastolic function, as recently reported in a comparison of hypertensive African Caribbeans and European whites drawn from the Anglo-Scandinavian Cardiac Outcomes (ASCOT) trial.[8] In African-Caribbean patients, echocardiographic studies revealed impaired diastolic function after adjustment for confounding variables, such as age, gender, systolic blood pressure, pulse pressure, cholesterol, smoking, ejection fraction (EF), left ventricular mass index, and diabetes mellitus (E': 7.52 vs 8.51; P <0.001; E/E': 8.89 vs 7.93; P=0.003; African Caribbeans vs white Europeans for both comparisons) (Figure 7-5). The finding of this study with respect to the association of left ventricular hypertrophy (LVF) and HF in people of African-American ancestry was consistent with those of the Third National Health and Nutrition Examination Survey (NHANES), which used electrocardiographic criteria to assess LVF.[9]

Therapeutic Considerations

Several studies have examined the optimum drug treatment for African Americans presenting with HF. The best known is the African-American Heart Failure Trial (A-HeFT), which was terminated early because of a significant survival benefit of fixed-dose combination isosorbide dinitrate plus hydralazine (BiDil®).[10] A subsequent extension to the same trial found that the benefits of this combination were sustained. It should be appreciated that these drugs were added against a background of optimum therapy with diuretics, digoxin, ACE inhibitors, and β-blockers.[11]

The effects of β-blockade with different doses of ACE inhibitors and digitalis were assessed in the Metoprolol CR/XL Randomized Intervention Trial in Congestive Heart Failure (MERIT-HF) in which patients with HF and left ventricular EF ≤40% were randomized to metoprolol CR/XL (Toprol-XL®) versus placebo.[12] Outcomes were analyzed separately for those on a low dose (≤median) of

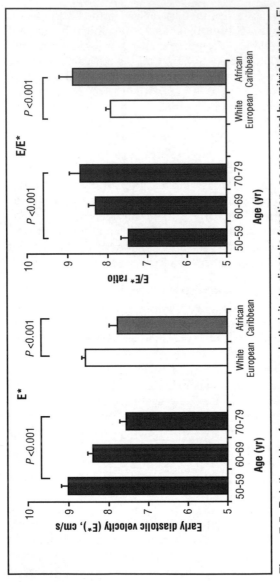

Figure 7-5: Relationship of age group and ethnicity to diastolic function, as measured by mitral annular E' and the E/E' ratio. The magnitude of the ethnic difference in these markers of diastolic function in comparison with that of each decade of aging is demonstrated. Diastolic function was assessed using the tissue Doppler early diastolic velocity (E') and the ratio of E' and the transmitral early filling velocity (E/E').[9]

the ACE inhibitors or digitalis versus high dose (>median). The mean dose of ACE inhibitors in the high-dose group (n=1,457) was 3 times higher than that in the low-dose group (n=2,094). Mortality was reduced to a similar extent in the high- and low-dose ACE inhibitor subgroups (relative risk [RR]=0.69 vs 0.64, respectively). Corresponding figures for combined mortality/all hospitalizations and for mortality/hospitalizations for HF were 0.85 versus 0.83, and 0.70 versus 0.68, respectively. Likewise, reduction in total mortality with metoprolol CR/XL was similar in patients receiving no digitalis (n=1,447; RR=0.56), low dose (n=1,122; RR=0.71), or high dose (n=1,421; RR=0.71). In a subsequent subgroup analysis, it has shown that this effect was also evident in African Americans.[13]

The Sudden Cardiac Death in Heart Failure (SCD-HeFT) trial demonstrated that implantable cardioverter/defibrillator (ICD) therapy significantly improved survival compared to medical therapy alone in stable, moderately symptomatic HF patients with an EF ≤35%. The outcomes in African Americans (17% of 2,521 subjects) were similar to those seen in whites despite having lower EF. A higher proportion of African Americans were designated as having nonischemic cardiomyopathy. Survival benefits from implantable ICD therapy in SCD-HeFT were not dependent on race. In addition, in this clinical trial there was no evidence that African Americans were less willing to accept ICD therapy than whites.[14]

Prevention of Heart Failure in African Americans

Hypertension is an important precursor to the development of HF in African Americans. The appropriate therapy for preventing progression to overt HF has been the subject of some debate because black and white patients may respond in different ways to the same therapeutic agent. A post hoc analysis of the 4,054 black and white participants of the Studies of Left Ventricular Dysfunction (SOLVD) prevention trial was undertaken to determine whether or not enalapril (Vasotec®) had comparable efficacy in asymptomatic left ventricular dysfunction (ALVD) in preventing the development of symptomatic HF in black and white patients.[15] The study found that randomization to enalapril was associated with a comparably significant reduction in the relative risk of the development of symptomatic HF in black (RR=0.67) and white patients (RR=0.61). Treatment with enalapril was also associated with a comparable reduction in the risk of the development of HF requiring medical therapy and in the composite end point of death or development of HF in black and white patients. Blacks with ALVD were at increased risk of the development of symptomatic HF (RR=1.81; 95% CI, 1.51-2.17, P <0.001) compared with whites, despite adjustment for available measures of disease severity. The researchers concluded that enalapril was equally efficacious in reducing the risk of progression of ALVD in the two ethnic groups.

However, the findings of the Antihypertensive and Lipid-Lowering Treatment to Prevent Heart Attack Trial (ALLHAT) appear to run counter to this recommendation. The metabolic syndrome is a common risk factor found in African Americans, and antihypertensive drugs with favorable metabolic effects are advocated for first-line therapy in hypertensive patients with the condition. Wright et al[16] performed a subgroup analysis of ALLHAT. This randomized, double-blind trial of 42,418 participants compared outcomes by race in hypertensive individuals with and without metabolic syndrome treated with four drug regimens: (1) a thiazide-type diuretic (chlorthalidone), (2) a calcium channel blocker (CCB) (amlodipine besylate), (3) an α-blocker (doxazosin mesylate), and (4) an ACE inhibitor (lisinopril). For the purpose of this study, the metabolic syndrome was defined as the presence of hypertension plus at least two of the following: fasting serum glucose level of at least 100 mg/dL, body mass index (BMI) calculated as weight in kg divided by height in m^2 of at least 30, fasting triglyceride (Tg) levels of at

Table 7-1: Relative Risk of Heart Failure Compared to Chlorthalidone (RR=1) (CI)

	Black	White
amlodipine	1.50 (1.18-1.90)	1.25 (1.06-1.47)
lisinopril	1.49 (1.17-1.90)	1.20 (1.01-1.41)
doxazosin	1.88 (1.42-2.47)	1.82 (1.51-2.19)

CI=confidence interval, RR=relative risk

least 150 mg/dL, and high-density lipoprotein cholesterol (HDL-C) levels of less than 40 mg/dL in men or less than 50 mg/dL in women. Significantly higher rates of HF were observed consistently across all treatment comparisons in those with the metabolic syndrome (Table 7-1).

Higher rates for combined cardiovascular disease were observed with lisinopril-chlorthalidone (RR, 1.24 [1.09-1.40] and 1.10 [1.02-1.19], respectively) and doxazosin-chlorthalidone comparisons (RR, 1.37 [1.19-1.58] and 1.18 [1.08-1.30], respectively) in black and nonblack participants with metabolic syndrome. Higher rates of stroke were seen in black participants only (RR, 1.37 [1.07-1.76] for the lisinopril-chlorthalidone comparison, and RR, 1.49 [1.09-2.03] for the doxazosin-chlorthalidone comparison). Black patients with metabolic syndrome also had higher rates of end-stage renal disease (RR, 1.70 [1.13-2.55]) with lisinopril compared with chlorthalidone. The major finding of this report was that, despite a more favorable metabolic profile, the CCB, ACE inhibitor, and α-blocker arms were not superior to the thiazide-type diuretic arm in preventing adverse clinical outcomes in hypertensive patients with the metabolic syndrome.

The ALLHAT findings, which failed to support the preference for CCBs, α-blockers, or ACE inhibitors compared with thiazide-type diuretics in patients with the metabolic syndrome, despite their more favorable metabolic profiles, was particularly true for black participants with metabolic syndrome. The magnitude of the excess risk of end-stage renal disease (ESRD 70%), HF (49%), and stroke (37%) and the increased risk of combined cardiovascular disease and combined coronary heart disease (CHD) strongly argue against the preference of ACE inhibitors over diuretics as the initial therapy in black patients with the metabolic syndrome. Similar higher risk was noted for those randomized to the α-blocker versus the diuretic.

It is also of interest that the recently published Diabetes REduction Assessment with ramipril and rosiglitazone Medication (DREAM) trial specifically designed to evaluate the effect of ACE inhibitor treatment in patients with impaired fasting glucose levels or impaired glucose tolerance reported no significant reduction in new-onset diabetes in participants randomized to ramipril compared with placebo.[17]

The consensus emerging from these studies in African Americans is that hypertension should be detected early and treated vigorously, initially with a thiazide diuretic together with lifestyle strategies such as exercise, weight management, and a reduction in sodium intake.[18]

American Indians

One of the largest studies that examined the prevalence of left ventricular dysfunction in middle-aged and older American Indians was the Strong Heart Study (SHS). In the second SHS examination, mild and severe left ventricular dysfunction was assessed in 3,184 American Indians by echocardiography (see Chapter 3 for details of study). Left ventricular dysfunction was categorized as mild (left ventricular ejection fraction [LVEF] 40%-54%) or severe

(EF <40%). Both mild and severe dysfunction were more common in men than in women (17.4% vs 7.2% and 4.7% vs 1.8%) and in diabetic than in nondiabetic participants (12.7% vs 9.1% and 3.5% vs 1.6%). On the basis of multivariate analyses, it was concluded that left ventricular dysfunction was present in approximately 14% of middle-aged to elderly American Indians and was independently associated with overt HF and CHD, male sex, hypertension, overweight, arterial stiffening, renal damage, and, less consistently, with older age and diabetes.[19]

This relatively high prevalence of HF in American Indians places a premium on early diagnosis. Okin et al[20] assessed the ability of the electrocardiographic strain pattern of ST depression (STD) and T-wave inversion in the lateral precordial leads to predict new HF in American Indians. Digital electrocardiograms were examined in 2,059 American-Indian participants in the second SHS examination with no history of HF. The absolute magnitude of ST segment deviation (STD) in leads V_5 and V_6 was measured using a computer-assisted system. During 5.7 +/-1.4 years of follow-up, HF developed in 77 participants (3.7%). Participants who developed HF had greater STD in leads V_5 and V_6 than those who did not. In univariate Cox analyses, STD was a significant predictor of new HF, with each 10-microV greater STD associated with a 31% greater risk of HF (hazard ratio [HR] 1.31, 95% confidence interval [CI] 1.24-1.39). In Cox multivariate analyses controlling for age, gender, diabetes, CHD, albuminuria, and other baseline risk factors, STD remained a significant predictor of incident HF (HR 1.22, 95%; CI 1.13-1.32 per 10-μV increment in STD; P <0.001). Presence of left ventricular wall motion abnormalities in the absence of clinical evidence of HF carried a hazard ratio of 3 for subsequent development of overt HF during an 8.5-year follow-up in the same population.[21] As expected from data in other subgroups in the US, the prevalence of HF was less common in women than in men.[22]

Conventional cardiovascular risk factors are also important considerations in planning preventive strategies for HF in American Indians. The available evidence suggests that particular attention should be paid to electrocardiographic changes and echocardiographic indices of diastolic dysfunction as potential markers for the development of overt HF.

Heart Failure in Hispanic and Chinese Populations

One of the few studies that has addressed the incidence of HF in ethnic Chinese and Hispanic populations is the Multi-Ethnic Study of Atherosclerosis (MESA—see Chapter 3 for details). A recent report from this study indicated that during a median follow-up of 4.0 years, 79 participants developed CHF (incidence rate: 3.1 per 1,000 person-years). Not surprisingly, African Americans had the highest incidence of CHF, followed by Hispanic, white, and Chinese-American participants (incidence rates: 4.6, 3.5, 2.4, and 1.0 per 1,000 person-years, respectively). Although risk of developing CHF was higher among African Americans compared with white participants (HR, 1.8), adding hypertension and/or diabetes mellitus to models including ethnicity eliminated statistical ethnic differences in incident HF. The incidence of HF in Hispanics was intermediate between African Americans and Caucasians and least in ethnic Chinese.[23] African Americans also had the highest proportion of incident HF not preceded by clinical MI (75%) compared with other ethnic groups (Figure 7-6), while an increase in left ventricular mass had the greatest effect among Hispanic and white participants.

An interesting facet of the management of HF is the impact of HF on the quality of life (QOL) in Hispanic populations. Health-related QOL was determined in a longitudinal study among white, black, and Hispanic adults with HF measured using the Minnesota Living with Heart

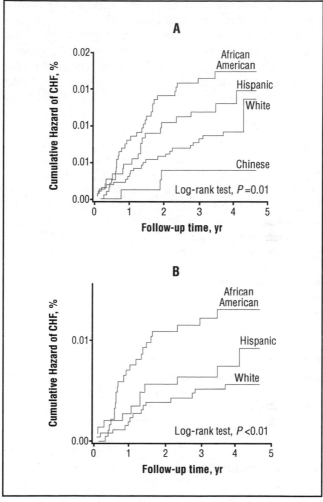

Figure 7-6: The risk of developing heart failure by ethnicity. (A) The risk is greatest in African Americans followed by Hispanics and least in ethnic Chinese. (B) The incidence of heart failure was not influenced by the occurrence of an MI during follow-up.[23]

Failure Questionnaire. It was observed that overall Hispanic patients compared with both black and white patients had more favorable scores, even after adjusting for baseline scores, age, gender, education, severity of illness, and care setting (acute vs chronic), and estimating the treatment effect (intervention vs usual care) compared to African Americans and Caucasians.[24]

South Asians

Data relating to HF are sparse in South-Asian populations (individuals originating primarily from India, Pakistan, Bangladesh, and Sri Lanka) living in the US. However, a retrospective analysis of hospital charts of patients with CHD completed in Canada showed an interesting trend.[25] South-Asian patients admitted with HF between 1997 and 1999 were significantly younger, had lower BMI, were more often diabetic, and were less often smokers than white counterparts. In-hospital mortality was not different between groups, although South Asians were more likely to experience ventricular arrhythmias. Despite presenting at a younger age, South Asians had more high-risk features at hospital discharge. Because South Asians are also at high risk of developing premature CAD (see Chapter 3), a more aggressive approach to prevention strategies in this ethnic group is indicated. A comparable study undertaken in a Health Service Trust in the United Kingdom also showed that South-Asian patients presenting with HF tended to be younger and had a higher prevalence of diabetes.[26]

Brown et al[27] conducted one of the few studies that addressed HF in Asians in the US. This study reviewed Medicare beneficiaries ≥65 years of age who were hospitalized in 2000 with a first-listed diagnosis of HF (International Classification of Diseases, 9th Revision, Clinical Modification code 428). They reported that prevalence of HF hospitalization increased over the 10-year period for white, black, Hispanic, and Asian enrollees, though one could not be certain of the exact origin of the Asian population. Prevalence was highest among those ≥85 years of age and the age-adjusted prevalence was greater among men than women. Compared with white enrollees in 2000, the likelihood of a HF hospitalization was 1.5 times greater among black enrollees, 1.2 times greater among Hispanic enrollees, and 0.5 times less likely among Asian enrollees after adjustment for age and sex (P <0.05 for all). Compared with white patients hospitalized with HF, black and Hispanic (but not Asian) patients were less likely than white patients to die in a hospital. A greater proportion of black, Hispanic, and Asian patients were discharged home than were white patients during 2000. Thus, the available evidence suggests that South Asians present at a younger age with HF, but their overall outlook seems more favorable than that of Caucasians.

A recent study addressed a possible genetic cause for development of HF in individuals from the Asian subcontinent.[28] It described a deletion of 25 base-pairs in the gene encoding cardiac myosin binding protein C (MYBPC3) that is associated with heritable cardiomyopathies and an increased risk of HF in Indian populations, which disrupts cardiomyocyte structure in vitro. Its prevalence was found to be high (~4%) in populations of Indian subcontinent ancestry. The finding of a common risk factor implicated in South-Asian subjects with cardiomyopathy will help in identifying and counseling individuals from this region predisposed to cardiac diseases.

Peripartum Cardiomyopathy

Peripartum cardiomyopathy is a rare disorder in which left ventricular dysfunction is diagnosed within the final month of pregnancy or within 5 months after delivery. It is a form of dilated cardiomyopathy in which no other cause of heart dysfunction can be identified. In the US, peripartum cardiomyopathy complicates 1 in every 1,300 to 4,000 deliveries. It may occur in childbearing women of any age, but it is most common after age 30. Risk factors include obesity, a personal history of cardiac disorders such as myocarditis, use of certain medications, smoking, alcoholism, multiple pregnancies, African-American ethnicity, and malnourished state.

The largest study of the incidence of peripartum cardiomyopathy in various ethnic minorities was performed in the Southern California Kaiser health-care system.[29] Between 1996 and 2005, there were 241,497 deliveries, and 60 cases of peripartum cardiomyopathy were identified on the basis of the following: (1) left ventricular EF <0.50, (2) met the Framingham criteria for HF, (3) occurrence of new symptoms of HF or initial echocardiographic diagnosis of left ventricular dysfunction before or within 5 months after delivery, and (4) absence of another discernible cause of HF. The overall incidence of peripartum cardiomyopathy was 1 in 4,025 deliveries. The incidence in whites, African Americans, Hispanics, and Asians was 1 of 4,075, 1 of 1,421, 1 of 9,861, and 1 of 2,675 deliveries, respectively. The incidence of peripartum cardiomyopathy was greatest in African Americans, which was 2.9-fold higher compared with whites ($P=0.03$) and 7-fold that of Hispanics ($P <0.001$). With a mean follow-up of 4.7 years, the freedom from all-cause death was 96.7% by the Kaplan-Meier method.

Novel Markers of Risk and HF

The influence of inflammatory markers and insulin resistance associated with the metabolic syndrome, albuminuria, and obesity on incident HF has been examined in the MESA study (see Chapter 3), which included men and women from four ethnicities: Caucasians, African Americans, Hispanics, and Chinese Americans who were followed for a median of 4 years.[30] Participants with a history of symptomatic CVD were excluded. Cox proportional hazards models were used to analyze the associations of the metabolic syndrome, inflammatory markers, insulin resistance, and albuminuria with incident HF, independent of established risk factors (age, gender, hypertension, diabetes mellitus, left ventricular hypertrophy, obesity, serum total cholesterol, and smoking), an interim MI, and baseline magnetic resonance imaging (MRI) parameters of left ventricular structure and function. Seventy-nine participants developed HF during follow-up, 26 participants (32.9%) had a prior MI, and 65% of the cases had preserved function (LVEF ≥40%). In multivariable analyses, serum interleukin-6 (IL-6), C-reactive protein (CRP), and macroalbuminuria were predictors of HF, independent of obesity and the other established risk factors. Although obesity was significantly associated with incident HF, this association was no longer significant after adding inflammatory markers (IL-6 or CRP) to the model. These findings suggest again that obesity and the metabolic syndrome should be addressed as therapeutic targets for prevention of HF.

References

1. Fauci AS, Longo DL, Braunwald E, et al: Heart failure and cor pulmonale. In *Harrison's Principles Of Internal Medicine*. 16th ed, vol 2. New York, NY, McGraw-Hill, 2005, pp 1367-1378.

2. Ravi K, Kappagoda T: Rapidly adapting receptors in acute heart failure and their impact on dyspnea. *Respir Physiol Neurobiol* 2009:167:107-115.

3. Uhley HN, Leeds SE, Sampson JJ, et al: Right duct lymph flow in experimental heart failure following acute elevation of left atrial pressure. *Circ Res* 1967;20:306-310.

4. National Heart, Lung, and Blood Institute: Data fact sheet. Congestive heart failure in the United States: a new epidemic. Accessed at: http://library.thinkquest.org/27533/facts.html.

5. Centers for Disease Control and Prevention: Fact Sheets and At–a–Glance Reports. Heart Failure Fact Sheet. 2010. Accessed at: http://www.cdc.gov/dhdsp/library/fs_heart_failure.html.

6. Loehr LR, Rosamond WD, Chang PP, et al: Heart failure incidence and survival (from the Atherosclerosis Risk in Communities study). *Am J Cardiol* 2008;101:1016-1022.

7.	Bibbins-Domingo K, Chertow GM, Fried LF, et al: Renal function and heart failure risk in older black and white individuals: The Health, Aging, and Body Composition Study. *Arch Intern Med* 2006;166:1396-1402.

8.	Sharp A, Tapp R, Francis DP, et al: Ethnicity and left ventricular diastolic function in hypertension. *JACC* 2008;52:1015-1021.

9.	Havranek EP, Froshaug DB, Emserman CD, et al: Left ventricular hypertrophy and cardiovascular mortality by race and ethnicity. *Am J Med* 2008;121(10):870-875.

10.	Taylor AL, Ziesche S, Yancy CW, et al: African-American Heart Failure Trial Investigators. Early and sustained benefit on event-free survival and heart failure hospitalization from fixed-dose combination of isosorbide dinitrate/hydralazine: consistency across subgroups in the African-American Heart Failure Trial. *Circulation* 2007;115:1747-1753.

11.	Yancy CW, Ghali JK, Braman VM: Evidence for the continued safety and tolerability of fixed-dose isosorbide dinitrate/hydralazine in patients with chronic heart failure (the Extension to African-American Heart Failure Trial). *Am J Cardiol* 2007;100:684-689.

12.	Ghali JK, Dunselman P, Waagstein F, et al: Consistency of the beneficial effect of metoprolol succinate extended release across a wide range dose of angiotensin-converting enzyme inhibitors and digitalis. *J Card Fail* 2004;10:452-459.

13.	Goldstein S, Deedwania P, Gottlieb S, et al: MERIT-HF Study Group. Metoprolol CR/XL in black patients with heart failure (from the Metoprolol CR/XL randomized intervention trial in chronic heart failure). *Am J Cardiol* 2003;92:478-480.

14.	Mitchell JE, Hellkamp AS, Mark DB, et al, and the SCD-HeFT Investigators: Outcome in African Americans and other minorities in the Sudden Cardiac Death in Heart Failure Trial (SCD-HeFT). *Am Heart J* 2008;155:501-506.

15.	Dries DL, Strong MH, Cooper RS, et al: Efficacy of angiotensin-converting enzyme inhibition in reducing progression from asymptomatic left ventricular dysfunction to symptomatic heart failure in black and white patients. *J Am Coll Cardiol* 2002;40:311-317.

16.	Wright JT Jr, Harris-Haywood S, Pressel S, et al: Clinical outcomes by race in hypertensive patients with and without the metabolic syndrome: Antihypertensive and Lipid-Lowering Treatment to Prevent Heart Attack Trial (ALLHAT). *Arch Intern Med* 2008;168:207-217.

17.   DREAM Trail Investigators, Dagenais GR, Gerstein HC, et al: Effects of ramipril and rosiglitazone on cardiovascular and renal outcomes in people with impaired glucose tolerance or impaired fasting glucose: results of the Diabetes REduction Assessment with ramipril and rosiglitazone Medication (DREAM) trial. *Diabetes Care* 2008;31:1007-1014.

18.   Svetkey LP, Simons-Morton D, Vollmer WM, et al: Effects of dietary patterns on blood pressure: subgroup analysis of the Dietary Approaches to Stop Hypertension (DASH) randomized clinical trial. *Arch Intern Med* 1999;159:285-293.

19.   Devereux RB, Roman MJ, Paranicas M, et al: A population-based assessment of left ventricular systolic dysfunction in middle-aged and older adults: the Strong Heart Study. *Am Heart J* 2001;141:439-446.

20.   Okin PM, Roman MJ, Lee ET, et al: Usefulness of quantitative assessment of electrocardiographic ST depression for predicting new-onset heart failure in American Indians (from the Strong Heart Study). *Am J Cardiol* 2007;100:94-98.

21.   Cicala S, de Simone G, Roman MJ, et al: Prevalence and prognostic significance of wall-motion abnormalities in adults without clinically recognized cardiovascular disease: The Strong Heart Study. *Circulation* 2007;116:143-150.

22.   Bella JN, Palmieri V, Roman MJ, et al: Gender differences in left ventricular systolic function in American Indians (from the Strong Heart Study). *Am J Cardiol* 2006;98:834-837.

23.   Bahrami H, Kronmal R, Bluemke DA, et al: Differences in the incidence of congestive heart failure by ethnicity. *Arch Intern Med* 2008;168(19):2138-2145.

24.   Riegel B, Moser DK, Rayens MK, et al: Heart Failure Trialists Collaborators. Ethnic differences in quality of life in persons with heart failure. *J Card Fail* 2008;14(1):41-47.

25.   Singh N, Gupta M: Clinical characteristics of South Asian patients hospitalized with heart failure. *Ethn Dis* 2005;15:615-619.

26.   Newton JD, Blackledge HM, Squire IB: Ethnicity and variation in prognosis for patients newly hospitalised for heart failure: a matched historical cohort study. *Heart* 2005;91:1545-1550.

27.   Brown DW, Shepard D, Giles WH, et al: Racial or ethnic differences in hospitalization for heart failure among elderly adults: Medicare, 1990 to 2000. *Am Heart J* 2005;150:448-454.

28.   Dhandapany PS, Sadayappan S, Xue Y, et al: A common MYBPC3 (cardiac myosin binding protein C) variant associated with cardiomyopathies in South Asia. *Nature Genetics* 2009;41:187-191.

29.   Brar SS, Khan SS, Sandhu GK, et al: Incidence, mortality, and racial differences in peripartum cardiomyopathy. *Am J Cardiol* 2007;100:302-304.

30.   Bahrami H, Bluemke DA, Kronmal R, et al: Novel metabolic risk factors for incident heart failure and their relationship with obesity: the MESA (Multi-Ethnic Study of Atherosclerosis) study. *J Am Coll Cardiol* 2008;51:1775-1783.

Chapter 8

Congenital Heart Defects

By Philip R. Liebson, MD

Congenital heart defects are found in approximately 1 in 125 newborns[1] and are associated with racial disparities in types, interventions, and mortality.[2] Although mortality from heart defects between 1979 and 1997 in the United States for all ages declined 39% (from 2.5 to 1.5 per 100,000 population)[2] and by a similar percentage for infants, mortality was 19% higher in blacks than in whites, 68.4 versus 55.5 per 100,000, respectively.[2] Infant mortality decreased considerably in this 18-year period for such major congenital heart defects as transposition of the great arteries, ventricular septal defect, atrioventricular septal defect, and aortic coarctation.[2] Moreover, although mortality decreased in blacks as well as in white infants, black infant mortality rates were consistently higher over this period.[2] In 1979, for example, infant deaths/100,000 were 107 for blacks and 96 for whites, and both rates decreased in a roughly parallel fashion, so that in 1997 those rates declined to 67/100,000 infant deaths for blacks and 54/100,000 infant deaths for whites.[2]

Overall, the average age of death increased for common congenital heart defects over the 18-year period but was higher in blacks. For all common congenital heart defects, between 1979-83 and 1994-97, the 50th percentile in mortality for whites increased from 7 months to 12 months, and for blacks only from 3 months to 5 months. For most anomalies, black mortality persisted at a younger age than whites for virtually all categories.[2] Categories in which deaths in blacks occurred at least half the age as whites or lower included ventricular septal defect, aortic valve and pulmonary valve anomalies, and single ventricle.

Lack of access to medical care, poor nutrition, and lack of maternal education may contribute to the development of neural tube defects.[3] Higher rates of neural tube defects were found in Hispanic women in Brooklyn than in black or non-Hispanic whites.[4] Racial variations in congenital defects varied widely among blacks and whites in a study from Atlanta, Georgia.[5] Congenital heart defects were found to be more common in American Indians in British Columbia than in the general population.[6] Fetal alcohol syndrome may be associated with congenital heart anomalies and the syndrome is particularly common in Native Americans, occurring in up to 103 of 100,000 live births.[7] On the basis of a population-based case control study of congenital cardiovascular malformations in Washington DC and the surrounding area between 1981-1987, birth weight deficits were found for infants with tetralogy of Fallot, endocardial cushion defect, hypoplastic left heart syndrome, pulmonary stenosis, coarctation of the aorta, and atrial and ventricular septal defects.[8]

An evaluation of congenital cardiac malformations by race and sex was evaluated in infants born in Louisiana in 1988-1989.[9] Variability included a significantly higher prevalence of atrioventricular canal defects per 1,000 live births in black females (0.74) compared with white females (0.41), black males (0.20), and white males (0.12). On the other hand, aortic stenosis and/or aortic coarctation were highest in white males. Single ventricle was higher in whites than blacks. Complete transposition of the great arteries was highest in white males (0.560) compared with black males (0.20), black females (0.17), and white females (0.12). These differences further demonstrated the variability of certain congenital cardiac defects by race and gender.

Table 8-1: Prevalence Rates of Congenital Heart Defects by Ethnic Group

Ethnic Group	Cases (no.)	Live Births (no.)	Prevalence[a] Rate	95% CI
Blacks	505	89,645	5.6[b]	5.1-6.1
Whites	1,654	230,363	7.2	6.8-7.5
Mexican Americans	350	59,553	5.9[b]	5.3-6.5

[a]Rate/1,000 live births

[b]Significantly (*P*<0.001) different from the rate in whites

CI=confidence interval

From Fixler[11] with permission from the American College of Cardiology © 1993.

A study of trends in Dallas County, Texas, in births from 1971-1984 found an overall prevalence rate of congenital heart malformations of 6.6/1,000.[10,11] The rate for whites, 7.2/1,000, was significantly higher than for Mexican Americans 5.9/1,000, or for blacks, 5.6/1,000 (Table 8-1).[11] Also, no differences were seen in the rates related to surgery, cardiac catheterization, or autopsy. Aortic stenosis, endocardial cushion defects, and ventricular septal defects had a higher prevalence in white infants and young children (Table 8-2).[11] The median age at diagnosis was similar among racial groups. In regard to socioeconomic variables and timing of referral to cardiologists, no significant differences were seen for family income or educational level of the parents.[11]

The first comprehensive estimates of leading congenital malformations among minority groups in the US were reported in 1988.[7] From 1981 to 1986, the Birth Defects

Table 8-2: Prevalence Rates[a] for Specific Heart Defects by Ethnic Group

Diagnostic Group	Blacks	
	Rate	No.
Ventricular septal defect	2.52[b]	226
Pulmonary stenosis	0.54	48
Atrial septal defect	0.38	34
Patent ductus arteriosus[c]	0.34	31
Endocardial cushion defect	0.21[b]	19
Aortic stenosis	0.07[d]	6
Coarctation	0.20	18
Tetralogy of Fallot	0.17	15
Hypoplastic left heart	0.24	22
d-Transposition	0.14	13

[a]Live born cases/1,000 live births.
[b]P <0.05 compared with rate in whites
[c]Excluding premature infants

Monitoring Program of the Centers for Disease Control and Prevention (CDC) found that Native Americans had the highest rates of atrial septal defect, valve stenosis and atresia, and fetal alcohol syndrome in regard to cardiac anomalies. Rates for patent ductus arteriosus and pul-

Whites		Mexican Americans	
Rate	No.	Rate	No.
3.04	700	2.55[b]	152
0.59	135	0.67	40
0.49	114	0.44	26
0.36	84	0.28	17
0.42	96	0.17[d]	10
0.40	92	0.20[b]	12
0.29	67	0.17	10
0.26	59	0.22	13
0.25	58	0.12	7
0.21	49	0.17	10

[d] P <0.005 compared with rate in whites

From Fixler[11] with permission from the American College of Cardiology © 1993.

monary stenosis were highest for blacks. Patent ductus arteriosus was the major cardiac congenital anomaly among blacks as well as Native Americans and Asians, frequently associated with high rates of prematurity. Down syndrome, commonly associated with ventricular septal defect, was most common for Hispanics, possibly related to advanced maternal age. Asians had the highest rates of ventricular septal defect.

The Metropolitan Atlanta Congenital Defects Program registry reported results from an evaluation of 5,813 major congenital heart defects between 1968 and 1997.[12] The overall prevalence was 6.2/1,000 live births, similar to other findings. However, the prevalence increased to 9.0/1,000 live births in the last two years of the evaluation.

The increase began in 1970 and was especially seen in the rising prevalence of ventricular septal defect, atrial septal defect, tetralogy of Fallot, and atrioventricular septal defect (Figure 8-1).[12] The reasons for this increase are unclear but may relate to increased availability of 2D echocardiography for diagnosis, especially in the case of less severe defects.

A higher overall occurrence of congenital heart defects was found in blacks compared with whites, primarily due to increased peripheral pulmonary stenosis and atrial septal defects. Temporal trends demonstrated an increase in overall rates of heart defects in both blacks and whites. Peripheral pulmonary stenosis increased more rapidly in blacks while ventricular septal defects and coarctation of the aorta increased more rapidly in whites.

The Texas Birth Defects Registry provided a report on records of children up to 1 year of age with aortic stenosis, coarctation of the aorta, or hypoplastic left heart syndrome born in 1999-2001.[13] These malformations were more common in males (7.7 vs 3.35/10,000 live births). Hispanic females had a similar prevalence compared with black and non-Hispanic white females.[13] Prevalence rates for Hispanic males were lower than for non-Hispanic white males (5.7), and lower for black males, even lower than the rate in black females (1.9 vs 3.5). Factors associated with increased congenital outflow defects included maternal age. Of environmental interest, increased prevalence of coarctation was found in the Texas-Mexican border compared with the rest of the state.

In terms of gender, death rates appear higher in boys, especially in infancy. Boys are more prone to have serious congenital heart conditions such as transposition of the great arteries, pulmonary and tricuspid atresia, aortic stenosis and coarctation of the aorta, and hypoplastic left heart syndrome. There is little information about the causes of racial disparities in mortality but recent studies shed some light on possible causes.

Risk Factors for Congenital Heart Defects

Environmental factors, which often vary among racial groups, may increase risk for congenital heart abnormalities. These include maternal rubella, phenylketonuria, diabetes, obesity, or exposure to pharmacologic agents such as ibuprofen, indomethacin, sulfasalazine, trimethoprim/sulfonamide and anticonvulsants.[14] Nontherapeutic drug exposure includes marijuana.

In regard to conditions in which racial minority groups may be particularly prone, pregestational diabetes may be associated with transposition of the great vessels, hypoplastic heart syndrome, patent ductus arteriosus, and looping defects in the fetus, to name but a few.[14] It has been suggested, based on animal model studies, that abnormal glucose levels in the mother leads to embryotoxic apoptotic cellular changes.[15]

Maternal obesity has been shown to have a 6-fold increased risk of aggregate cardiac defects among black women (OR 6.5; 95% CI 1.2-34.9; P=0.025).[16] Maternal alcohol consumption during the first trimester of pregnancy and marijuana use have been associated with ventricular septal defects.[17] Recent studies have variably found an association between maternal smoking and congenital defects, including atrial septal defects, atrioventricular septal defects, and tetralogy of Fallot.[18]

However, black infants appear to have a lower incidence of many congenital heart defects compared with white infants. In the Baltimore-Washington Infant Study, a popula-

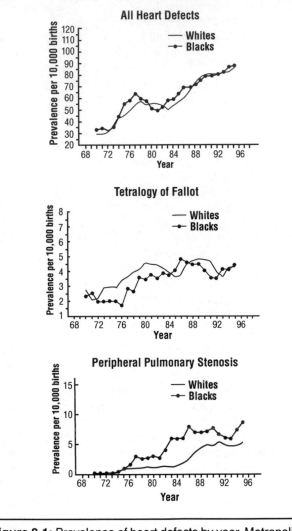

Figure 8-1: Prevalence of heart defects by year, Metropolitan Atlanta, 1968-1997. Prevalence is based on 10,000 births and is presented as a 5-year moving average.

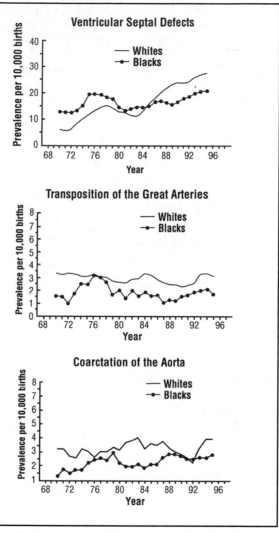

From Botto[12] with permission from the American Academy of Pediatrics © 2001.

tion-based study of 2,087 cases of congenital malformations, an excess of white infants were found with aortic stenosis, atrioventricular septal defects, atrial septal defects, coarctation, patent ductus arteriosus, and tetralogy of Fallot.[7,19] Pulmonary stenosis was more common in black infants. Controlling for socioeconomic status disclosed a white excess for L-transposition of the great arteries. Aortic stenosis was limited to low- and middle-income strata.[19] However, in a population-based study, the prevalence of birth defects in infants of black and Hispanic women showed no significant variation compared with infants from non-Hispanic white women.[20]

Genetic Considerations

A large number of chromosomal disorders have been associated with congenital heart disease.[21] A population-based study of the 22q11.2 deletion in Atlanta between 1994-1999 found an increased frequency among Hispanics compared with whites, blacks, and Asians.[22] This chromosomal abnormality is associated with increased congenital anomalies, especially right aortic arch and interrupted aortic arch, and tetralogy of Fallot.

Mortality, Results of Interventions, and Insurance Issues

Mortality risk variations in congenital heart defect surgery among racial groups may be influenced by unequal access to care. This was explored in a population-based cohort study using hospital discharge data from four states (California, Massachusetts, New York, and Pennsylvania) in 1996.[23] Surgical mortality was lower in whites than in nonwhites (3.7% vs 5.1%, $P=0.02$). Unadjusted mortality rates varied among Asian, Hispanic, black and "other" groups (5.3%, 4.9%, 4.1%, 7.3%, respectively, $P=0.008$). When adjusted for risk factors, Asians and Hispanics still had a higher risk of dying from surgery than did non-Hispanic whites, but not blacks. Variations appeared between states. For example, blacks had a higher risk of dying compared to whites in Massachusetts but a lower risk in Pennsylvania.[24,25]

In a study of California hospital discharges after surgical repair for congenital heart disease in patients <18 years of age in 1995-1996, patients with private insurance were younger than those with managed care insurance plans (Figure 8-2).[24] Asians tended to be older than other racial groups but only significantly for ventricular septal defects. Native Americans were excluded from this as well as other studies mentioned because of small sample sizes.

Considerations of racial disparities in outcomes may be associated with recommendations for surgery related to insurance coverage. For example, pediatric heart surgery in those with managed care insurance was found to be less likely accomplished in lower mortality hospitals than children who were covered by commercial insurance.[14,26,27]

In an evaluation of the timing of just two complex palliative procedures that require surgery early in life, bidirectional Glenn and Fontan stages of single ventricle palliation at the Duke University Medical Center, black children underwent the Glenn procedure at a median age of 11 months compared to 5 months for whites.[28] Black children underwent the Fontan procedure at a median of 60 months, white children at 36 months.

The influence of insurance coverage on mortality after congenital heart disease surgery was further evaluated in a retrospective cohort study using hospital discharge data from five stated between 1992 and 1996.[27] In 1996, children with Medicaid, more commonly covering minority racial groups, had a higher risk of death than those with commercial or managed care insurance. Moreover, Medicaid patients had a higher risk of death than those with commercial insurance at both higher and lower mortality institutions. It is possible that children covered by Medicaid are referred later to a pediatric cardiologist. Other considerations for higher postsurgical mortality among minority groups are

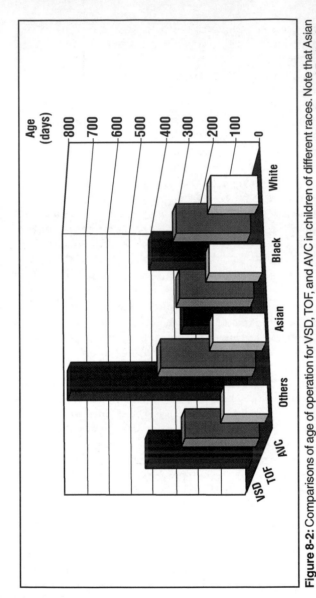

Figure 8-2: Comparisons of age of operation for VSD, TOF, and AVC in children of different races. Note that Asian children tended to be older at surgery. From Chang[24] with permission from the American Academy of Pediatrics © 2000. AVC=atrioventricular septal defects, TOF=tetralogy of Fallot, VSD=ventricular septal defects.

Table 8-3: Effects of Race/Ethnicity on Mortality After Congenital Heart Surgery, Adjusted for Baseline Risk, Gender, Income, and Geographic Region

Race/Ethnicity	OR	95% CI	P
White	1.00	-	-
Black	1.76	(1.23, 2.52)	0.002
Hispanic	1.34	(1.00, 1.81)	0.05
Asian	0.82	(0.48, 1.38)	NS

Adapted from Benavidez[28] with permission from Springer Science + Business Media, Inc. © 2006.

language barriers that prevent patients from reporting symptoms earlier, lack of regular checkups in Medicaid groups, poor prenatal care, and intra-uterine growth retardation.[27] From a database of 2,784 institutions in 27 states, a more recent analysis of racial and ethnic disparities in mortality following congenital heart surgery was investigated.[28] As in previous analyses, black children had a higher death rate than whites (OR 1.65, P=0.003) (Table 8-3).[28] Hispanic children had an insignificantly higher death rate than non-Hispanic whites. Adjustment for gender, income, and region continued to demonstrate a significantly higher postsurgical mortality in blacks (OR 1.76) but also in Hispanics (OR 1.34) compared with non-Hispanic whites. In this evaluation, insurance did not appear to play a role in gender differences, although blacks and Hispanics had higher rates of Medicaid insurance (56% each) compared with non-Hispanic whites (23%). Although Medicaid patients exhibited a trend toward higher mortality in unadjusted analyses, this difference was minimal after adjustment for risk factors. This lack of insurance impact compared with previous analyses may have been due to statewide children's health-care programs of more recent vintage, or the more comprehensive national study in this case.

Significant regional variations were seen in mortality risk for blacks but not Hispanics. For example, only in the Northeast was mortality risk higher for blacks versus whites, and was not significantly increased in other regions.

In summary, racial differences in congenital heart defect mortality generally, and surgical mortality specifically, may be caused by a combination of genetic and environmental factors. These could include differences in prenatal care affecting intrauterine growth and development, disproportionate variations in the prevalence of diabetes, age of the mother, differences in medical training of physicians caring for diverse racial groups, differences in mortality rates in hospitals serving minority groups, language barriers, and other factors that affect access to acceptable medical care.

As with other aspects of cardiovascular disease in special groups, better access to medical care and focus on risk factor interventions need to be accomplished to decrease such disparities in outcome.

References

1. National Heart, Lung and Blood Institute: Congenital heart defects. December 2007. Accessible at: www.nhlbi.nih.gov/health/dci/Diseases/chd/chd_what.html. Accessed June 16, 2009.

2. Boneva RS, Botto LD, Moore CA, et al: Mortality associated with congenital heart defects in the United States. Trends and racial disparities, 1979-1997. *Circulation* 2001;103;2376-2381.

3. Windham GC, Ednmonds LD: Current trends in incidence of neural tube defects. *Pediatrics* 1982;70:333-337.

4. Feldman JG, Stein SC, Klein RJ, et al: The prevalence of neural tube defects among ethnic groups in Brooklyn, New York. *J Chronic Dis* 1982;35:53-60.

5. Erickson JD: Racial variations in the incidence of congenital abnormalities. *Ann Hum Genet* 1976;39:315-320.

6. Lowry RB, Thunem NY, Silver M: Congenital anomalies in American Indians in British Columbia. *Genet Epidemiol* 1986;3:455-467.

7. Chavez GF, Cordero JF, Becerra JE: Leading major congenital malformations among minority groups in the United States, 1981-1986. *MMWR Surveillance Summaries* 1988;37(SS-3);17-24.

8. Rosenthal GL, Wilson PD, Permutt T, et al: Birth weight and cardiovascular malformations: a population-based study. The Baltimore-Washington Infant Study. *Am J Epidemiol* 1991; 133:1273-1281.

9. Storch TG, Mannick EE: Epidemiology of congenital heart disease in Louisiana: an association between race and sex and the prevalence of specific cardiac malformations. *Teratology* 1992;46:271-276.

10. Fixler DE, Pastor P, Chamberlin M, et al: Trends in congenital heart disease in Dallas County births, 1971-1984. *Circulation* 1990;81:137-142.

11. Fixler DE, Pastor P, Sigman E, et al: Ethnicity and socioeconomic status: impact on the diagnosis of congenital heart disease. *J Am Coll Cardiol* 1993;21:1722-1726.

12. Botto LD, Correa A, Erickson JD: Racial and temporal variations in the prevalence of heart defects. *Pediatrics* 2001;107:E2-8.

13. McBride KL, Marengo L, Canfield M, et al: Epidemiology of noncomplex left ventricular outflow tract obstruction malformations (aortic valve stenosis, coarctation of the aorta, hypoplastic left heart syndrome) in Texas, 1999-2001. *Birth Defects Research (Part A)* 2005;73:555-561.

14. Jenkins KJ, Correa A, Feinstein JA, et al: Noninherited risk factors and congenital cardiovascular defects: Current knowledge. A scientific statement from the American Heart Association Council on Cardiovascular Disease in the Young. *Circulation* 2007;115:2995-3014.

15. Phelan PA, Ito M, Loeken MR: Neural tube defects in embryos of diabetic mice: role of Pax-3 gene and apoptosis. *Diabetes* 1997;46:1189-1197.

16. Mikhail LN, Walker CK, Mittendorf R: Association between maternal obesity and fetal cardiac malformations in African Americans. *J Natl Med Assoc* 2002;04:695-700.

17. Tikkanen J, Heinonen OP: Risk factors for ventricular septal defect in Finland. *Public Health* 1991;105:99-112.

18. Torfs CP, Christianson RE: Maternal risk factors and major associated defects in infants with Downs's syndrome. *Epidemiology* 1999;10:264-270.

19. Correa-Villaseñor A, McCarter R, Downing J, et al: White-black differences in cardiovascular malformations in infancy and socioeconomic factors. The Baltimore-Washington Infant Study Group. *Am J Epidemiol* 1991;134:393-402.

20. Carmichael, SL, Nelson V, Shaw GM, et al: Socioeconomic status and risk of conotruncal heart defects and orofacial clefts. *Paediatric Perinatal Epidemiol* 2003;17:264-271.

21. Pierpont ME, Barron CT, Benson TW Jr, et al: Genetic basis for congenital heart defects: current knowledge. A scientific statement from the American Heart Association Congenital Cardiac Defects Committee, Council on Cardiovascular Disease in the Young. *Circulation* 2007;115:3015-3038.

22. Botto LD, May K, Fernhoff PM, et al: A population-based study of the 22q11.2 deletion: Phenotype, incidence, and contribution to major birth defects in the population. *Pediatrics* 2003;112:101-107.

23. Gonzalez PC, Gauvreau K, De Mone JA, et al: Regional racial and ethnic differences in mortality for congenital heart surgery in children may reflect unequal access to care. *Pediatr Cardiol* 2003; 24:103-108.

24. Chang RK, Chen AY, Klitzner TS: Factors associated with age at operation for children with congenital heart disease. *Pediatrics* 2000;105:1073-1081.

25. Milazzo AS Jr, Sanders SP, Armstrong BE, et al: Racial and geographic disparities in timing of bidirectional Glenn and Fontan stages of single-ventricle palliation. *J Natl Med Assoc* 2002;94:873-878.

26. Erickson LC, Wise PH, Cook EF, et al: The impact of managed care insurance on use of lower-mortality hospitals by children undergoing cardiac surgery in California. *Pediatrics* 2000;105:1271-1278.

27. DeMone JA, Gonzalez PC Gauvreau K, et al: Risk of death for Medicaid recipients undergoing congenital heart surgery. *Pediatr Cardiol* 2003;24:97-102.

28. Benavidez OJ, Gauvreau K, Jenkins KJ: Racial and ethnic disparities in mortality following congenital heart surgery. *Pediatr Cardiol* 2006;27:321-328.

Chapter 9

Metabolic Factors and Coronary Heart Disease

By C. Tissa Kappagoda, MD, PhD
and Ezra A. Amsterdam, MD

The main metabolic factors that have an impact on coronary heart disease (CHD) are obesity, the metabolic syndrome, and diabetes mellitus. The prevalence of each has increased steadily over the past two decades in the United States.

Obesity

Obesity has a significant adverse impact on several risk factors for CHD.[1] Overweight and obesity are both labels for ranges of weight that exceed what is considered healthy for a given height. The first federal guidelines on the identification, evaluation, and treatment of overweight and obesity were released in 1997 by the National Heart, Lung, and Blood Institute, in cooperation with the National Institute of Diabetes and Digestive and Kidney Diseases.[2] Approximately 97 million adults in the US are overweight or obese, both of which increase the risk of a number of diseases, including hypertension; dyslipidemia; type 2 diabetes; CHD; stroke; gallbladder disease; osteoarthritis; sleep apnea and respiratory problems; and endometrial, breast, prostate, and colon cancers. Additionally, higher body weights are associated with increased all-cause mortality.

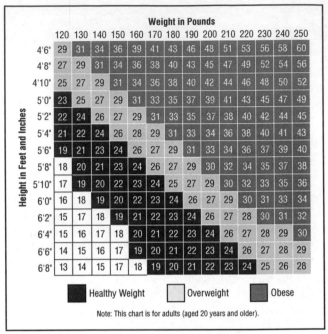

Figure 9-1: Body mass index (BMI) chart (Source: US Surgeon General). Accessible at: https://vic.pvhs.org/pls/portal/docs/page/pvhs/pvhs_document_mgmt2/doc_services/services%20gastric%20bypass%20sg_bmi_table.pdf)

The measure that is generally accepted for evaluating an individual's weight in terms of its impact on health is the body mass index (BMI) (Figure 9-1). The formula for computing BMI is:

BMI = weight (kg)/height (m²); the ranges for BMI are listed in Table 9-1.

These recommended classifications may vary periodically and depend on the ethnicity of the population under consideration. However, despite its wide acceptance, BMI

Table 9-1: Ranges of Body Mass Index (kg/m²)

	Males	Females
Underweight	<20	<18
Normal	≥20 to <25	≥18 to <23
Overweight	≥25 to <30	≥23 to <30
Obese	≥30	≥30
Morbidly obese	>35	>35

does not always present an accurate picture of these issues in special populations. For example, it is recommended that the normal/overweight threshold for Southeast Asian body types be lowered to a BMI of 23.[3] The new cut-off BMI for obesity in Asians is 27.5 compared with the traditional figure of 30 defined by the World Health Organization (WHO). An Asian adult with a BMI of 23 or greater is now considered overweight, and the ideal normal range is 18.5–22.9. Application of current Western criteria for both the metabolic syndrome and BMI may lead to an underestimation of conditions such as the metabolic syndrome in Asians living in the US.[4]

The BMI could potentially convey significant errors in estimating health in people who are lean because it tends to overestimate obesity (and by implication body fat). A recent meta-analysis has shown that abdominal obesity as determined by the waist–hip ratio is a significantly better predictor of multiple cardiovascular diseases (CVD) such as hypertension, hyperlipidemia, and type 2 diabetes than is BMI.[5] Also, in an analysis of 40 studies involving 250,000 people with pre-existing coronary artery disease, those with normal BMIs were at higher risk of death from CVD than were people with BMIs in the overweight range.[6]

During the past 20 years, the US has seen a dramatic increase in obesity (Figure 9-2). In 2007, only one state (Colorado) had a prevalence of obesity <20%. Thirty states had a prevalence equal to or greater than 25% and in three of these states (Alabama, Mississippi, and Tennessee) the prevalence of obesity was ≥30%.[7]

Metabolic Syndrome

The metabolic syndrome has been recognized as a clinical entity in one form or another for more than 80 years and has at times been termed the deadly quartet, syndrome X, plurimetabolic syndrome, the insulin resistance syndrome, and the dysmetabolic syndrome.[8] The National Cholesterol Education Program Adult Treatment Panel III (NCEP ATP III) defines the condition based on the presence of three of the following factors: abdominal obesity, elevated serum triglycerides (Tg), low levels of high-density lipoprotein (HDL), hypertension, and elevated blood glucose. As detailed in the ATP III report, participants having three or more of the following criteria were defined as having the metabolic syndrome:

(a) Abdominal obesity: waist circumference >102 cm in men and >88 cm in women;

(b) Hypertriglyceridemia: Tg ≥150 mg/dL (1.69 mmol/L);

(c) Low levels of HDL-cholesterol (HDL-C): <40 mg/dL (1.04 mmol/L) in men and <50 mg/dL (1.29 mmol/L) in women;

(d) Hypertension: ≥130/85 mm Hg;

(e) High fasting glucose: glycosylated hemoglobin (HbA$_{1c}$) ≥110 mg/dL (≥6.1 mmol/L).

The fasting glucose value has been the subject of much debate. The American Association of Clinical Endocrinologists (AACE) has recommended a range of 110 to 126 mg/dL, while the American Diabetes Association (ADA) has suggested a value of >100 mg/dL.[9] Regardless of the actual cut point for hyperglycemia, it is the *clustering*

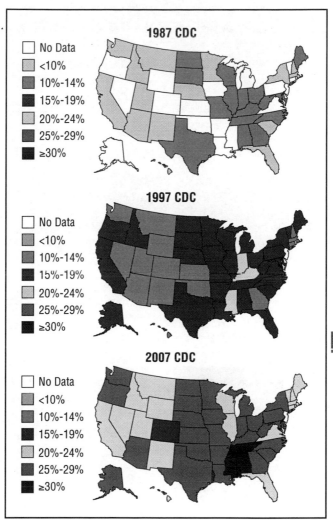

Figure 9-2: Prevalence of obesity by states in the US: 1987, 1997, and 2007. Prevalence is defined as the percentage of people with a body mass index greater than 30. Accessible at: http://www.cdc.gov/nccdphp/dnpa/obesity/trend/maps/

Table 9-2: Three Definitions of the Metabolic Syndrome

WHO Criteria (1999)	European Group for the Study of Insulin Resistance (1999)
Diabetes, impaired fasting glycemia, impaired glucose tolerance or insulin resistance, plus	Insulin resistance, plus
2 of the following:	*2 of the following:*
Obesity: BMI >30 or waist-to-hip ratio >0.9 (male) and >0.85 (female)	*Central obesity:* Waist circumference ≥37 in (male) or 31.5 in (female)
Dyslipidemia: Triglycerides >150 mg/dL or HDL <35 mg/dL (male) and <40 mg/dL (female)	*Dyslipidemia:* Triglycerides >175 mg/dL or HDL <40 mg/dL
Hypertension: Blood pressure >140/90 mm Hg	*Hypertension:* Blood pressure ≥140/90 mm Hg with or without medications
Microalbuminuria: Excretion >20 μg/min	*Fasting plasma glucose:* >100 mg/dL

WHO=World Health Organization; BMI=body mass index; NCEP III=National Cholesterol Education Program Adult Treatment Panel III; HDL=high-density lipoprotein

NCEP III (2001)

3 of the following:

Central obesity:

Waist circumference ≥40 in (male)
or 35 in (female)

Dyslipidemia:

Triglycerides >150 mg/dL or

HDL <40 mg/dL (male)
and <45 mg/dL (female)

Hypertension:

Blood pressure ≥135/85 mm Hg
with or without medications

Fasting plasma glucose:

>110 mg/dL

of these factors that demands consideration as a specific syndrome because of its impact on CHD. Furthermore, these factors, when viewed as individual entities, do not usually engage the attention of physicians in a manner that would lead to effective therapy. The definitions of the syndrome by WHO and the European Group for the Study of Insulin Resistance (EGIR) also differ slightly from the previously mentioned definitions (Table 9-2), but do not appear to influence the indications for treatment required for patients with this condition.

The Third National Health and Nutrition Examination Survey III, 1988-1994 (NHANES III), based on a cross-sectional health survey of a nationally representative sample of the noninstitutionalized civilian US population (8,814 men and women 20 years of age or older), provided the first estimate of prevalence of the metabolic syndrome in the US, as defined in the ATP III report. The unadjusted and age-adjusted prevalences of the metabolic syndrome were 21.8% for men and 23.7%, for women. The prevalence increased from 6.7% among participants 20 to 29 years of age to 43.5% and 42.0% for those 60 to 69 years of age and 70 years, respectively (Figure 9-3). Based on 2000 census data, about 47 million US residents have the metabolic syndrome. The highest prevalence was found in Hispanic-American women and the lowest in African-American men (Figure 9-4).[10]

A total of 6,436 men and women ≥20 years of age from NHANES III and 1,677 participants from NHANES (1999-2000) were included in a second analysis to determine the changes in prevalence of the metabolic syndrome in the US. Once again, the ATP III definition of the metabolic syndrome was used in this analysis.[11] The unadjusted prevalence of the metabolic syndrome was 23.1% for the group from NHANES III and 26.7% in NHANES 1999-2000 (P=0.043), and the age-adjusted prevalences were 24.1% and 27.0% (P=0.088), respectively. The age-adjusted prevalence increased by 23.5% among women (P=0.021)

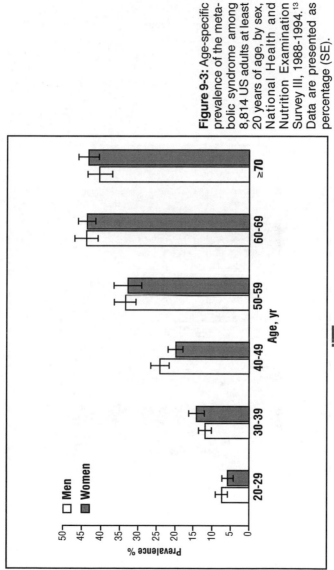

Figure 9-3: Age-specific prevalence of the metabolic syndrome among 8,814 US adults at least 20 years of age, by sex, National Health and Nutrition Examination Survey III, 1988-1994.[13] Data are presented as percentage (SE).

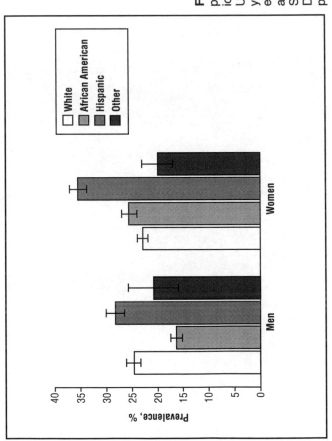

Figure 9-4: Age-adjusted prevalence of the metabolic syndrome among 8,814 US adults aged at least 20 years, by sex and race, or ethnicity, National Health and Nutrition Examination Survey III, 1988-1994.[13] Data are presented as percentage (SE).

and 2.2% among men ($P=0.831$). Increases in hypertension, waist circumference, and hypertriglyceridemia accounted for much of the rise in the prevalence of the metabolic syndrome, particularly among women. In particular, the prevalence of this syndrome escalated rapidly among women 20 to 39 years of age. Large increases in the prevalences of hypertriglyceridemia and hypertension were largely responsible for the increase among women. The authors concluded that the increased prevalence of the metabolic syndrome was likely to lead to future increases in diabetes and CVD.

Diabetes Mellitus

From 1980 through 2005, the number of Americans with diabetes increased from 5.6 million to 15.8 million. People ≥65 years of age account for approximately 38% of the population with diabetes. In general, the prevalence of confirmed diabetes was higher for blacks and Hispanics than for whites across all age groups. Regardless of race/ethnicity and sex, prevalence tended to be highest among persons ≥65 years of age and lowest among persons <45 years of age.[12]

In these surveys, all sampled adults were asked whether or not a health professional had ever told them they had diabetes. To exclude gestational diabetes, women were asked whether or not they had been told they had diabetes other than during pregnancy. Also, parents of sampled children were asked whether or not their child had diabetes. Three-year averages were used to improve the precision of the annual estimates. Also, prevalence of diabetes was estimated by age, race, ethnicity, and sex. *However, persons of Hispanic origin were deemed to be of any race.*

Metabolic Issues in African Americans
Obesity

The prevalence of obesity among African Americans is comparable to that in Caucasian populations. There has also

Table 9-3: Changes in Age-Adjusted Prevalence of Obesity and Extreme Obesity by Sex and Racial/Ethnic Group for Adults Aged 20 Years and Older*

Sex	Racial/Ethnic Group	NHANES III, 1988-1994 No.	NHANES III, 1988-1994 % (SE)
Both sexes	All*	16,681	22.9 (0.68)
Men	All*	7,933	20.2 (0.72)
	Non-Hispanic white	3,285	20.3 (0.85)
	Non-Hispanic black	2,112	21.1 (1.02)
	Mexican American	2,250	23.9 (0.97)
Women	All*	8,748	25.4 (0.95)
	Non-Hispanic white	3,755	22.9 (1.15)
	Non-Hispanic black	2,490	38.2 (1.37)
	Mexican American	2,128	35.3 (1.36)

NHANES=National Health and Nutrition Examination Survey; CI=confidence interval

*Includes racial/ethnic groups not shown separately

**Does not meet the standard of statistical reliability and precision (relative SE >30%)

Obesity (BMI ≥30)

	NHANES, 1999-2000	
No.	% (SE)	Change, % (95% CI)
4,115	30.5 (1.43)	7.6 (4.4 to 10.8)
2,043	27.5 (1.61)	7.3 (3,8 to 10.8)
946	27.3 (1.82)	7.0 (3.0 to 11.0)
374	28.1 (2.27)	7.0 (2.0 to 12.0)
538	28.9 (2.25)	5.0 (0.1 to 9.9)
2,072	33.4 (1.81)	8.0 (3.9 to 12.1)
885	30.1 (2.10)	7.2 (2.4 to 12.0)
420	49.7 (2.79)	11.5 (5.3 to 17.7)
567	39.7 (3.65)	4.4 (-3.4 to 12.2)

9

Table 9-3: Changes in Age-Adjusted Prevalence of Obesity and Extreme Obesity by Sex and Racial/Ethnic Group for Adults Aged 20 Years and Older* *(continued)*

Sex	Racial/Ethnic Group
Both sexes	All*
Men	All*
	Non-Hispanic white
	Non-Hispanic black
	Mexican American
Women	All*
	Non-Hispanic white
	Non-Hispanic black
	Mexican American

NHANES=National Health and Nutrition Examination Survey; CI=confidence interval

*Includes racial/ethnic groups not shown separately

**Does not meet the standard of statistical reliability and precision (relative SE >30%)

Extreme Obesity (BMI ≥40)

NHANES III, 1988-1994, % (SE)	NHANES, 1999-2000, % (SE)	Change, % (95% CI)
2.9 (0.23)	4.7 (0.56)	1.8 (0.6 to 3.0)
1.7 (0.32)	3.1 (0.58)	1.4 (0.1 to 2.7)
1.8 (0.41)	3.0 (0.75)	1.2 (-0.5 to 2.9)
2.4 (0.38)	3.5 (1.24)**	1.1 (-1.5 to 3.7)
1.1 (0.33)**	2.4 (0.74)**	1.3 (-0.3 to 2.9)
4.0 (0.31)	6.3 (0.78)	2.3 (0.6 to 4.0)
3.4 (0.40)	4.9 (0.89)	1.5 (-0.5 to 3.5)
7.9 (0.51)	15.1 (2.05)	7.2 (3.0 to 11.4)
4.8 (0.65)	5.5 (1.04)	0.7 (-1.8 to 3.2)

been a significant increase in its prevalence over the last 10 years, as shown by successive NHANES surveys. The current prevalence of obesity in Caucasians, African Americans, and Hispanics is approximately 28% (Table 9-3). In this analysis, obesity was defined as a BMI ≥30 kg/m^2.[13]

Metabolic Syndrome

Multiple studies have addressed the metabolic syndrome in African Americans, one of the most compelling of which is NHANES III. Metabolic syndrome-associated factors and prevalence, as defined by ATP III criteria, were evaluated in a representative US sample of 3,305 black, 3,477 Mexican-American, and 5,581 white men and nonpregnant or nonlactating women ≥20 years of age. The metabolic syndrome was present in 22.8% and 22.6% of US men and women, respectively (P=0.86). The age-specific prevalence was highest in Mexican Americans and lowest in blacks of both sexes. Ethnic differences persisted even after adjusting for age, BMI, and socioeconomic status (Figure 9-4). Findings similar to NHANES III were obtained in the Atherosclerosis Risk in Communities (ARIC) baseline survey, in 1987 through 1989.[14]

However, recent data from the Jackson Heart Study (JHS) point to a more disturbing trend among African Americans with respect to the metabolic syndrome.[15] Among those 35 to 84 years of age who were recruited at baseline during 2000 through 2004, the metabolic syndrome prevalence was 43.3% in women and 32.7% in men after diabetics were excluded. Elevated blood pressure (70.4%), abdominal obesity (64.6%), and low HDL-C (37.2%) were highly prevalent. Prevalence rates for CVD, CHD, and cerebrovascular disease (CBD) were 12.8%, 8.7%, and 5.8%, respectively. After adjustment for age and sex, the metabolic syndrome was associated with increased age. The authors concluded that the prevalence of the metabolic syndrome in this group was among the highest reported for population-based cohorts worldwide and was significantly

Table 9-4: Age-Related Prevalence of the Metabolic Syndrome in African Americans (Jackson Heart Study) [15]

	Subjects (n)	Metabolic syndrome (%)
Age (P_{diff})		<0.0001
Overall	4,706	39.4
21–34 years	236	16.5
35–44 years	911	25.4
45–54 years	1,169	36.4
55–64 years	1,277	48.2
65–74 years	845	50.2
75–84 years	244	45.5
85+ years	15	33.3
Sex (P_{diff})		<0.0001
Female	2,998	43.3
Male	1,708	32.7

9

associated with increased odds ratios for CVD, CHD, and CBD. A high prevalence of low HDL emerged as a leading contributor to the metabolic syndrome among African Americans in this large cohort (Table 9-4).

Diabetes

The ARIC cohort[16] provided definitive data showing that the prevalence of diabetes mellitus is higher in African Americans than in the general population. A total of 2,646 African-American and 9,461 white adults, 45 to 64 years of age without diabetes at baseline, were sampled from four US communities. Incident type 2 diabetes, ascertained by self-report of physician diagnosis, use of diabetes medications, or fasting glucose level of at least 7.0 mmol/L (126 mg/dL) were compared among white and African-American subjects and by presence of potentially modifiable risk factors. Diabetes incidence per 1,000 person-years was about 2.4-fold greater in African-American women and about 1.5-fold greater in African-American men than in their white counterparts ($P < 0.001$) (Table 9-5). Results from proportional hazards regression models indicated that racial differences in potentially modifiable risk factors, particularly adiposity, accounted for 47.8% of the excess risk in African-American women, but for little excess risk in African-American men. Compared with their white counterparts, African-American men and women had higher blood pressure before diabetes onset (diastolic blood pressure difference=5.6 mm Hg in women and 8.4 mm Hg in men; P=0.005). The authors concluded that middle-aged African Americans are at greater risk of developing type 2 diabetes and have higher blood pressure prior to development of diabetes. In women, almost 50% of this excess risk might be related to *potentially modifiable factors*.

A recent analysis of African Americans who developed diabetes has yielded additional information about risk factors for CVD in the ARIC cohort.[17] In 741 African Americans 45 to 64 years of age with diabetes, 143 developed CVD. Risk factors were measured from 1987 through 1998. The crude incidence rate (per 1,000 person-years) of CVD was 22.5 (11.9 for CHD and 12.0 for stroke). After multivariate adjustments, total cholesterol, prevalent hypertension, and current smoking were significantly and positively associated with incident CVD among these African Americans with diabetes (Table 9-5). Among the nonconventional risk factors, serum creatinine, factor VIII, von Willebrand factor, and white blood cell count were positively and independently associated with CVD incidence, while serum albumin was negatively and independently associated with CVD incidence. Adjusted relative risks for highest versus lowest tertiles of these risk factors

Table 9-5: Incident Type 2 Diabetes Mellitus in 12,107 Adults With No Evidence of Diabetes at Baseline[18]

	Women		Men	
	African American	White	African American	White
No. of persons	1,690	5,093	976	4,368
Person years of follow up	11,873	40,911	6,891	34,102
Incident cases of diabetes	298	425	161	541
Incidence/1,000 person-years	25.1	10.4	23.4	15.9
(Confidence interval)	(22.4-28.1)	(9.4-11.4)	(19.9-27.2)	(14.6-17.2)

9

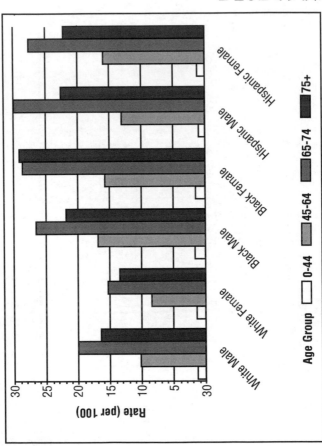

Figure 9-5: Age-specific prevalence of diagnosed diabetes, by race/ethnicity, and sex, US, 2005. Accessible at:http://www.cdc.gov/diabetes/statistics/prev/national/figpersons.htm

ranged from 1.77 to 2.13. This study again confirmed that the major risk factors (hypercholesterolemia, hypertension, and smoking) were important determinants of CVD in African Americans with diabetes. In addition, several blood markers of hemostasis or inflammatory response and elevated serum creatinine also proved to be risk factors for CVD in African Americans with diabetes.

Hispanics

The prevalence of obesity among Hispanics is similar to that in African Americans and Caucasians (Table 9-3).[13] Bearing in mind the problems discussed in Chapter 3, relating to establishing ethnicity in populations designated nominally as Hispanic, a significant body of evidence suggests that the prevalences of both the metabolic syndrome and diabetes are higher among Hispanics (Figures 9-4 and 9-5). The prevalence of diabetes in people ≥20 years of age, after adjusting for age differences in the population in the National Health Interview Survey (2004-2006), showed the following ethnic distribution:

- 6.6% of non-Hispanic whites
- 7.5% of Asian Americans
- 10.4% of Hispanics
- 11.8% of non-Hispanic blacks

Among Hispanics the rates were:
- 8.2% for Cubans
- 11.9% for Mexican Americans
- 12.6% for Puerto Ricans.

American Indians

American Indians are particularly disadvantaged in terms of their propensity to develop CHD. Over the last two decades a significant body of information derived mainly from the Strong Heart Study has provided a basis for considering them to be a unique population. Diabetes and hypertension appear to be particularly important risk factors in this group. The prevalence of obesity and the metabolic syndrome is also high and the latter is a strong indicator for developing overt diabetes and CHD over a 10-year period.[18] The Indian Health Service (IHS) population database, which includes data for approximately 1.4 million American Indians and Alaska Natives in the US who receive health care from the IHS, shows that 14.2% of the American Indians and Alaska Natives ≥20 years of age had diagnosed diabetes. After adjusting for population age differences, 16.5% of the total adult population served by the IHS had diagnosed diabetes, with rates varying by region from 6.0% among Alaska-Native adults to 29.3% among American-Indian adults in southern Arizona.

Thus, in assessing American Indians, even asymptomatic individuals should be screened proactively for the metabolic syndrome, peripheral arterial disease (PAD), and early evidence of renal dysfunction in the form of microalbuminuria and proteinuria.

Specific Metabolic Issues Pertaining to CHD in Minorities
C-Reactive Protein (CRP)

High sensitivity C-reactive protein (hs-CRP) is an acute-phase reactant largely produced by the liver in response to inflammatory cytokines such as interleukin-6 (IL-6) that has been viewed as an inactive downstream marker of low-grade vascular inflammation. It is considered the best available risk predictor, and the American Heart Association (AHA) recommends its measurement to further risk stratify individuals at intermediate risk (10%-20% 10-year risk) for heart disease. In low-risk individuals, its value is debatable. Much of the controversy resides in the population being studied. In older men and women, for instance, elevated CRP was independently associated with increased 10-year risk of CHD.[19] The authors claimed that "a single CRP measurement provided information beyond conventional risk assessment, especially in intermediate-Framingham-risk men and high-Framingham-risk women." Such sweeping generalizations should be viewed with caution because the male population studied was >65 years of age, and according to the NCEP III scheme for assessment of global risk, such individuals are already almost in the high-risk category on the basis of their gender and age. Furthermore, the biological variation in a single estimate of CRP in an individual has a coefficient of variation of >100%.[20,21]

While the association between CRP levels and risk is recognized, although with some reservations, interpretation of specific values may depend on both gender and ethnicity. The Multiethnic Study of Atherosclerosis (MESA) addressed this issue in its cohort of 6,814 men and women 45 to 84 years of age (see Chapter 3).[22] After adjustment for other conventional risk factors, women had substantially higher median CRP levels compared with men (2.56 vs 1.43 mg/L, P <0.0001). These differences were evident even after adjusting for estrogen usage and BMI. The pattern of higher CRP levels in women was consistent across all ethnic subgroups after multivariable adjustment, and it was suggested that specific cut points for CRP should be employed for risk stratification.

The results of the Dallas Heart Study provided additional support for these findings. The CRP status was measured in 2,749 white and black subjects 30 to 65 years of age.[23] African-American subjects had higher CRP levels than white subjects (median, 3.0 vs 2.3 mg/L; P <0.001), and women had higher CRP levels than men (median, 3.3 vs 1.8 mg/L; P <0.001). The proportion of subjects with CRP levels >3 mg/L was 31%, 40%, 51%, and 58% in white men, black men, white women, and black women, respectively (P <0.05 for each group vs white men). After adjustment for traditional cardiovascular risk factors, estrogen and statin use, and BMI, a CRP level >3 mg/L remained more common in both white and black women. It was not known whether or not these gender and ethnic differences were predictive of future cardiovascular events. In addition, in the Women's

9

Health Study (WHS), median CRP levels were significantly higher among black women (2.96 mg/L, interquartile range [IQR] 1.19-5.86) than among their white (2.02 mg/L, IQR 0.81- 4.37), Hispanic (2.06 mg/L, IQR 0.88-4.88), and Asian (1.12 mg/L, IQR 0.48-2.25) counterparts. These differences could not be explained by the use of hormone replacement therapy (HRT) and other conventional risk factors.[24] Presentation of data in the form of interquartile changes implied that 25% of the data is in excess of the upper value, providing additional support for the significant variability associated with the measurement.

In 2008, Arima et al[25] investigated the effects of hs-CRP on the risks of CHD in a general population of Japanese. This was a prospective cohort study of 2,589 participants ≥40 years of age who were followed for 14 years. The median CRP level was 0.43 mg/L at baseline. During the follow-up period, 129 coronary events (myocardial infarction [MI], coronary revascularization, and sudden cardiac death) were observed. Age- and sex-adjusted annual incidence rates of CHD rose progressively with higher CRP levels: 1.6, 3.3, 4.5, and 7.4 per 1,000 person-years for quartile groups defined by CRP levels of <0.21, 0.21 to 0.43, 0.44 to 1.02, and >1.02 mg/L, respectively (P <0.0001 for trend). The risk of CHD in the highest quartile group was 2.98-fold (95% CI, 1.53-5.82) higher than that in the lowest group, even after controlling for other cardio-vascular risk factors. The authors concluded that hs-CRP levels were clearly associated with future CHD events in a general population of Japanese. However, in the Japanese populations, the CRP cut-off point for high risk of future development of CHD was >1.0 mg/L, which is much lower than that for Western populations.

Thus, it could be argued that concentrations of CRP should be interpreted with reference to ethnicity and gender. Additional support for this view is provided by the evidence that CRP levels in blood are a heritable characteristic in Japanese Americans.[26]

226

A recent study found that the distribution of genotypes and alleles in a Chinese-Han population was significantly different from that of the Caucasian population. There were no significant differences between frequencies of genotype and alleles of controls and those of patients ($P > 0.05$), but in controls the concentrations of CRP in the CC genotype subgroup were significantly higher than those in the CT genotype subgroup ($P < 0.05$). This observation suggests that the +1444C/T variant in the CRP gene could influence the basal CRP level in normal people. Thus, it may be necessary to establish genotype-specific risk thresholds of the CRP level as well.[27] While it is accepted that CRP levels in blood are correlated with CHD, it is likely that these potential genetic influences call for a more nuanced interpretation of the cut points, especially in women.[28]

The MESA has shown that CRP levels could also predict left ventricular failure in individuals without evident heart failure or other cardiovascular disorders. Higher CRP was associated with lower systolic myocardial function in all regions in men, but not in women. These findings support the role of inflammation and atherosclerosis in incipient myocardial dysfunction.[29] The Strong Heart Study showed that a combination of ST segment depression in the resting electrocardiogram and CRP increases the risk of mortality (all-cause and cardiovascular disease) in American Indians, demonstrating the additive impact of active inflammation and preclinical CVD on prognosis.[30]

Salt Sensitivity

It has been widely recognized since the 1960s that the prevalence of hypertension is significantly higher among African Americans than in their Caucasian counterparts. Many researchers have sought explanations for this finding, citing observations that suggested that African Americans have an exaggerated blood pressure response to salt loading. It has been hypothesized that this phenomenon might be traced to selective mortality during the period of Atlantic slavery.[31] Central to this hypothesis is the view that a genetic predisposition to retain sodium afforded protection during the rigors of excessive electrolyte loss associated with a physically demanding sea voyage. This hypothesis further reasons that this effect could be maladaptive in descendents living in the current high sodium environment. This concept has become known as the "Slavery hypothesis" and is intimately linked to its primary proponent, Clarence Grim. The hypothesis has been attacked robustly by both historians[32] and epidemiologists,[33] primarily on the grounds that there is no "smoking gun" in the form of a salt-retaining gene in African Americans. In the absence of alternative conventional sources of information, such as contemporary medical records relating the illnesses among the reluctant voyagers, the historical dimensions of the issue are likely to remain unresolved.

Despite these potentially contentious issues, African Americans do exhibit a sensitivity to salt in terms of blood pressure. In normotensive black men but not white men, salt sensitivity occurs when dietary potassium is even marginally deficient but is dose-dependently suppressed when dietary potassium is increased within its normal range. Such suppression might prevent or delay the occurrence of hypertension, particularly in many blacks whose dietary potassium is deficient. In one study,[34] 38 healthy normotensive men (24 blacks, 14 whites) were given a basal diet low in sodium (15 mmol/d) and marginally deficient in potassium (30 mmol/d) and then salt loaded (250 mmol/d). Throughout the last 3 weeks, potassium was supplemented (as potassium bicarbonate) to either mid- or high-normal levels (70 and 120 mmol/d). With moderate levels of potassium intake, salt loading increased blood pressure in African Americans—an effect not evident at higher intakes of potassium.[34] Also, correlations of blood pressure with aldosterone were more consistent and more striking in blacks than in French Canadians, while there were inconsistent correlations of blood pressure with atrial natriuretic factor in both ethnic groups. These observations are consistent with the hypothesis that aldosterone-induced volume expansion is an important contributor to hypertension, especially in blacks.[35]

Recent studies have examined the heritability of salt sensitivity in African Americans. Both hypertensive and normotensive adults were phenotyped with respect to salt sensitivity with an intravenous (IV) sodium-loading, furosemide volume-depletion protocol, and it was shown that salt sensitivity was likely to be a heritable characteristic.[36] Genes encoding adrenergic receptors are candidate loci for the inheritance of this hypertension-related trait because of the role of these receptors in the regulation of renal sodium excretion and vascular tone. Svetkey et al[37] studied hypertensive black American probands and their first-, second-, and third-degree relatives. Both hypertensive and normotensive siblings were tested for salt sensitivity by an IV sodium-loading, Lasix® volume-depletion protocol (ie, by the change in blood pressure under the two conditions). Genotyping was performed with restriction fragment length polymorphisms in genomic DNA probed with clones containing the β_2- and α_2-c10-adrenergic receptor genes. A total of 109 sib pairs were evaluated. Systolic pressure decreased by an average of 9.0 +/- 9%, diastolic pressure by 1.5 +/- 11%, and mean arterial pressure by 5.0 +/- 9%. Neither blood pressure nor salt sensitivity was linked at the α_2-c10-adrenergic receptor locus. No evidence suggested that salt sensitivity and baseline systolic blood pressure were linked at the β_2-adrenergic receptor locus. The diastolic blood pressure response to sodium loading/volume depletion was linked to the β_2-adrenergic receptor locus.

The genes associated with the renin-angiotensin system were examined in African Americans and Hispanics in the MESA cohort.[38] Examiners observed no significant increase

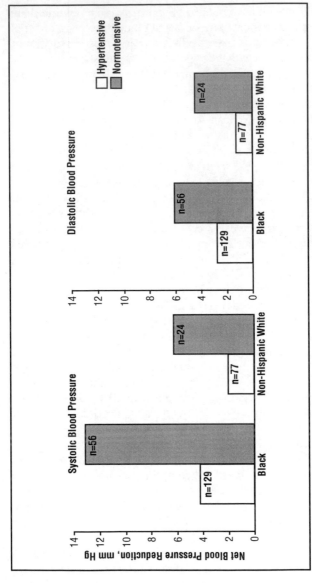

Figure 9-6: Effect of the DASH diet on systolic and diastolic blood pressure in whites and blacks.[39]

in the risk of hypertension for either African Americans or Hispanics homozygous or heterozygous for the D allele of the angiotensin-converting enzyme (ACE) gene. However, among African Americans, those who were carriers of the (-344)T allele of CYP11B2 were at increased risk of hypertension. There was also an increase in risk of hypertension associated with the AGTR1 T allele for African Americans. The associations observed with CYP11B2 and AGTR1 genotypes were not observed among Hispanics.

At a practical level, the Dietary Approaches to Stop Hypertension (DASH) provided additional information about African Americans in relation to the management of hypertension. In this randomized, controlled feeding study, 459 adults were fed a control diet for 3 weeks and then randomized to 8 weeks of (a) control diet; (b) a diet rich in fruits and vegetables; or (c) a combination diet rich in fruits, vegetables, and low-fat dairy foods, and reduced in saturated fat, total fat, and cholesterol (the DASH combination diet). Weight and salt intake were held constant. The combination diet lowered systolic blood pressure significantly more in African Americans (6.8 mm Hg) than in whites (3.0 mm Hg) (Figure 9-6).[39]

Taken collectively, these investigations in African Americans suggest that there may have been an unintended element of selection in the enforced voyage to the New World.

References

1.   Eckel RH, for the Nutrition Committee: Obesity and heart disease: a statement for healthcare professionals from the Nutrition Committee, American Heart Association. *Circulation* 1997;96:3248-3250.

2.   National Institutes of Health: Obesity. 1997. Accessible at: http://hp2010.nhlbihin.net/oei_ss/download/pdf/CORESET1.pdf.

3.   World Health Organization Expert Consultation: Appropriate body-mass index for Asian populations and its implications for policy and intervention strategies. *Lancet* 2004;363:157-163.

4.   Enas EA, Mohan V, Deepa M, et al: The metabolic syndrome and dyslipidemia among Asian Indians: a population with high rates of diabetes and premature coronary artery disease. *J Cardiometab Syndr* 2007;2:267-275

5.   Lee CM, Huxley RR, Wildman RP, et al: Indices of abdominal obesity are better discriminators of cardiovascular risk factors than BMI: a meta-analysis. *J Clin Epidemiol.* 2008;61:646-653.

6.   Romero-Corral A, Montori VM, Somers VK, et al: Association of bodyweight with total mortality and with cardiovascular events in coronary artery disease: a systematic review of cohort studies. *Lancet* 2006;368:666-678.

7.   Centers for Disease Control and Prevention: Obesity maps. 2007. Accessible at: http://www.cdc.gov/nccdphp/dnpa/obesity/trend/maps/. Accessed May 26, 2009.

8.   Kappagoda CT, Amsterdam EA: Management of patients with the metabolic syndrome: Compliance or adherence to treatment? In Krentz and Wong, eds. *Metabolic Syndrome and Cardiovascular Disease.* New York, Informa Healthcare, 2007.

9.   Grundy SM, Brewer HB, Cleeman JI, et al, for the Conference Participants Definition of Metabolic Syndrome: Report of the National Heart, Lung, and Blood Institute/American Heart Association Conference on Scientific Issues Related to Definition. *Circulation* 2004;109:433-438.

10.   Ford ES, Giles WH, Dietz WH: Prevalence of the metabolic syndrome among US adults: findings from the Third National Health and Nutrition Examination Survey. *JAMA* 2002;287:356-359.

11.   Ford ES, Giles WH, Mokdad AH: Increasing prevalence of the metabolic syndrome among U.S. Adults. *Diabetes Care* 2004;27:2444-2449.

12.   Centers for Disease Control and Prevention: Diabetes data and trends, 2008. Accessed February 2, 2010, at: http://www.cdc.gov/diabetes/statistics/prev/national/figpersons.htm.

13.   Flegal KM, Carroll MD, Ogden CL, et al: Prevalence and trends in obesity among US adults, 1999-2000. *JAMA* 2002;288:1723-1727.

14.   Schmidt MI, Duncan BB , Watson RL, et al: A metabolic syndrome in whites and African-Americans. The Atherosclerosis Risk in Communities baseline study. *Diabetes Care* 1996;19:414-418.

15. Taylor H, Liu J, Wilson G, et al: Distinct component profiles and high risk among African Americans with metabolic syndrome: the Jackson Heart Study. *Diabetes Care* 2008;31:1248-1253.

16. Brancati FL, Kao WH, Folsom AR, et al: Incident type 2 diabetes mellitus in African American and white adults: the Atherosclerosis Risk in Communities Study. *JAMA* 2000;283:2253-2259.

17. Adeniyi A, Folsom AR, Brancati FL, et al: Incidence and risk factors for cardiovascular disease in African Americans with diabetes: the Atherosclerosis Risk in Communities (ARIC) study. *J Natl Med Assoc* 2002;94:1025-1035.

18. de Simone G, Devereux RB, Chinali M, et al, Strong Heart Study Investigators: Prognostic impact of metabolic syndrome by different definitions in a population with high prevalence of obesity and diabetes: the Strong Heart Study. *Diabetes Care* 2007;30: 1851-1856.

19. Cushman M, Arnold AM, Psaty BM, et al: C-reactive protein and the 10-year incidence of coronary heart disease in older men and women: the cardiovascular health study. *Circulation* 2005;112: 25-31.

20. Macy EM, Hayes TE, Tracy RP: Variability in the measurement of C-reactive protein in healthy subjects: implications for reference intervals and epidemiological applications. *Clin Chem* 1997;43:52-58.

21. Ali N, Michikazu S, Sadanobu K: Intra-individual variability of high-sensitivity C-reactive protein: age-related variation over time in japanese subjects. *Circulation*;70:559-563.

22. Lakoski SG, Cushman M, Criqui M, et al: Gender and C-reactive protein: data from the Multiethnic Study of Atherosclerosis (MESA) cohort. *Am Heart J* 2006;152:593-598.

23. Khera A, McGuire DK, Murphy SA, et al: Race and gender differences in C-reactive protein levels. *J Am Coll Cardiol* 2005;46(3): 464-469.

24. Albert MA, Glynn RJ , Buring J, et al: C-reactive protein levels among women of various ethnic groups living in the United States (from the Women's Health Study). *Am J Cardiol* 2004;93:1238-1242.

25. Arima H, Kubo M, Yonemoto K, et al: High-sensitivity C-reactive protein and coronary heart disease in a general population of Japanese: the Hisayama study. *Arterioscler Thromb Vasc Biol* 2008;28:1385-1391.

26. Austin MA, Edwards KL, McNeely MJ, et al: Heritability of multivariate factors of the metabolic syndrome in nondiabetic Japanese Americans. *Diabetes Care* 2004;53:1166-1169.

27. Yan M, Zhao L, Zheng F, et al: The relationship between gene polymorphism and CRP level in a Chinese Han population. *Biochem Genet* 2007;45:1-9.

28. Crawford DC, Sanders CL, Qin X, et al: Genetic variation is associated with C-reactive protein levels in the Third National Health and Nutrition Examination Survey. *Circulation* 2006;114: 2458-2465.

29. Rosen BD, Cushman M, Nasir K, et al: Relationship between C-reactive protein levels and regional left ventricular function in asymptomatic individuals: the Multi-Ethnic Study of Atherosclerosis. *J Am Coll Cardiol* 2007;49:594-600.

30. Okin PM, Roman MJ, Best LG, et al: C-reactive protein and elec-trocardiographic ST-segment depression additively predict mortality: the Strong Heart Study. *J Am Coll Cardiol* 2005;45:1787-1793.

31. Wilson TW, Grimm CE: Biohistory of slavery and blood pressure differences in blacks today: a hypothesis. *Hypertension* 1991;17:122-128.

32. Curtin, PD: The slavery hypothesis for hypertension among African Americans: The historian evidence. *Am J Public Health* 1992;82:1681-1686.

33. Cooper RS, Kaufman JS Ward R: Race and genomics. *N Engl J Med* 2003;348:1166-1170.

34. Morris RC Jr, Sebastian A, Forman A, et al: Normotensive salt sensitivity: effects of race and dietary potassium. *Hypertension* 1999;33:18-23.

35. Grim CE, Cowley AW, Hamet P, et al: Hyperaldosteronism and hypertension ethnic differences. *Hypertension* 2005;45(4): 766-772.

36. Svetkey LP, McKeown SP, Wilson AF: Heritability of salt sensitivity in black Americans. *Hypertension* 1996;28:854-858.

37. Svetkey LP, Chen YT, McKeown SP, et al: Preliminary evidence of linkage of salt sensitivity in black Americans at the beta 2-adren-ergic receptor locus. *Hypertension* 1997;29:918-922.

38. Henderson SO, Haiman CA, Mack W: Multiple polymorphisms in the renin-angiotensin-aldosterone system (ACE, CYP11B2,

AGTR1) and their contribution to hypertension in African Americans and Latinos in the multiethnic cohort. *Am J Med Sci* 2004;288:266-273.

39. Svetkey LP, Simons-Morton D, Vollmer WM, et al: Effects of dietary patterns on blood pressure: subgroup analysis of the Dietary Approaches to Stop Hypertension (DASH) randomized clinical trial. *Arch Intern Med* 1999;159:285-293.

Chapter 10

Heart Disease in the Elderly

By C. Tissa Kappagoda, MD, PhD,
and Ezra A. Amsterdam, MD

The number of Americans 65 years of age and older will more than double to 71 million by 2030, comprising roughly 20% of the United States population. In some states, fully a quarter of the population will be 65 years of age and older. The cost of providing health care for an older American is three to five times greater than the cost for someone younger than 65 years of age. By 2030, the nation's health-care spending is projected to increase by 25% because of these demographic shifts, unless improving and preserving the health of older adults are more actively addressed.[1] For the purposes of this chapter, the term "older" includes people 65 years of age or greater.

As the US grows more diverse, so does the elderly population. In 2003, older Americans were 83% non-Hispanic white, 8% black, 6% Hispanic, and 3% Asian. By 2030, an estimated 72% of older Americans will be non-Hispanic white, 11% Hispanic, 10% black, and 5% Asian. Higher levels of education, which are linked to better health, higher income, more wealth, and a higher standard of living in retirement will continue to increase among the elderly. The proportion of Americans with at least a bachelor's degree grew five-fold from 1950 to 2003, from 3.4% to 17.4%, and by 2030, more than one quarter of the older population is expected to have an undergraduate degree. The percentage completing high school quadrupled between 1950 and 2003, from 17.0% to 71.5%. Substantial educational differences by race and Hispanic origin exist, despite the overall rise in educational attainment within the older population. In 2003, 76% of older non-Hispanic whites, 70% of older Asians, 52% of older blacks, and 36% of older Hispanics had completed high school. The gender gap for persons completing college will narrow in the future because men and women in younger cohorts are earning college degrees at roughly the same rate,[2] with recent data indicating that women are actually surpassing men in this pursuit.

These trends are likely reflected in the prevalence of heart disease in the elderly population. Although the age-adjusted death rates for heart disease declined in the US from 1990 to 2002 by approximately 24% (27% for men and 23% for women),[3] the number of individuals with these diseases will increase because of the rise in the aging population.

Serum Lipids

Studies of the association between cholesterol and mortality by race and ethnicity in the elderly have been inconsistent. For example, the Evans County Health Study[4] found a J-shaped relationship of cholesterol with all-cause mortality among white men but not in black men, and an inverse association between total cholesterol and all-cause mortality among African-American women but not in white women. Serum cholesterol levels were not related to all-cause or coronary heart disease (CHD) mortality among black men or white women. A recent report from a *free-living* multiethnic cohort of northern Manhattan Medicare recipients contained similar findings.[5] The cohort consisted of 2,556 nondemented elderly (65-103 yr: 66.1% women, 27.6% white/non-Hispanic, 31.2% African American, and 41.2% Hispanic).

In terms of all-cause mortality, Hispanics had the best overall survival, followed by African Americans and whites (Figure 10-1). Whites and African Americans in the lowest quartiles of total cholesterol, non-high-density lipoprotein

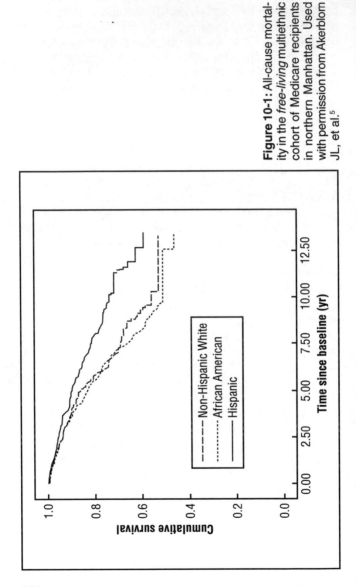

Figure 10-1: All-cause mortality in the *free-living* multiethnic cohort of Medicare recipients in northern Manhattan. Used with permission from Akerblom JL, et al.[5]

238

cholesterol (non-HDL-C), and low-density lipoprotein cholesterol (LDL-C) were approximately twice as likely to die as those in the highest quartile (Tables 10-1 and 10-2). In contrast, plasma lipid levels were not related to mortality risk among Hispanics. The effects of total cholesterol, non-HDL-C, and LDL-C were similar among white and African-American elders, despite a higher prevalence of hypertension, diabetes, and current smoking among African Americans. Hispanic participants, who had the highest prevalence of hypertension, diabetes, stroke, and dementia, showed the lowest all-cause mortality risk. No correlation was found between all-cause mortality and plasma lipid levels. Results were similar in analyses using ethnic group-specific cut points for quartiles of lipid levels or using cut points generated from the overall sample, suggesting that these findings are robust.

Similar conclusions were drawn from another study, also from the northern Manhattan area, where it was found that nondemented elderly individuals with levels of total cholesterol, non-HDL-C, and LDL-C in the lowest quartile were approximately twice as likely to die as those in the highest quartile (rate ratio [RR]=1.8, 95% confidence interval [CI]=1.3-2.4). These results did not vary when analyses were adjusted for body mass index (BMI), apolipoprotein E genotype, diabetes mellitus, heart disease, hypertension, stroke, cancer diagnosis, current smoking status, or demographic variables. The authors concluded that low cholesterol level is a robust predictor of mortality in the nondemented elderly and may be a surrogate of frailty or subclinical disease.[6]

Akerblom et al[5] have argued in favor of the so-called Hispanic paradox in the elderly. One possible explanation they have advanced is that of a healthy survivor. The mean age of their sample was 77 at baseline. Subjects with higher lipid levels and with high risk of acute cardiovascular events possibly died prior to recruitment, and the sample represents a group of healthy survivors with traits that make them less susceptible to disease caused by high lipid levels.

Table 10-1: Baseline Characteristics in the North Manhattan Elderly Cohort

Characteristics	Caucasian
Sample size, n (%)	705 (27.6)
Age at baseline, mean ± SD	77.3 ± 6.9
Sex[a]	
Male, n (%)	271 (38.4)
Female, n (%)	434 (61.6)
Age at baseline, mean ± SD	77.3 ± 6.9
Education, mean ± SD[a]	13.0 ± 3.5
BMI, mean ± SD	26.5 ± 5.1
C (mg/dL), mean ± SD	202.3 ± 38.5
HDL (mg/dL), mean ± SD[a]	47.8 ± 14.8
Tg (mg/dL), mean ± SD[a]	157.3 ± 84.5
LDL (mg/dL), mean ± SD	123.1 ± 32.6
Heart disease, n (%)[a]	211 (31.2)
Hypertension, n (%)[a,b]	354 (52.4)
Diabetes, n (%)[a,b]	80 (11.9)
Stroke, n (%)[b]	60 (8.9)
Dementia, incident, n (%)[a]	28 (4.0)
Currently smoking, n (%)[a]	59 (8.4)
Not currently smoking, n (%)[a]	646 (91.6)

[a]$P < 0.05$

[b]Numbers are less than 2,556 due to missing data

BMI=body mass index, C=cholesterol, HDL=high-density lipoprotein, LDL=low-density lipoprotein, SD=standard deviation, Tg=triglycerides

African American	Hispanic	Total Cohort
797 (31.2)	1,054 (41.2)	2,556 (100)
77.2 ± 6.5	76.6 ± 6.4	77.0 ± 6.6
250 (31.4)	346 (32.8)	867 (33.9)
547 (68.6)	708 (67.2)	1,689 (66.1)
77.2 ± 6.5	76.6 ± 6.4	77.0 ± 6.6
10.9 ± 3.8	6.7 ± 4.3	9.7 ± 4.8
27.8 ± 6.3	27.7 ± 5.1	27.4 ± 5.5
200.5 ± 38.0	198.4 ± 41.1	200.1 ± 39.6
51.9 ± 16.0	44.5 ± 13.7	47.7 ± 15.1
129.4 ± 67.9	176.0 ± 94.7	156.3 ± 86.5
122.7 ± 34.2	118.7 ± 36.0	121.2 ± 34.6
161 (21.0)	220 (21.8)	592 (24.2)
524 (68.5)	717 (71.3)	1,595 (65.2)
168 (21.9)	260 (25.8)	508 (20.7)
84 (11.0)	121 (12.0)	265 (10.8)
96 (12.1)	177 (16.8)	301 (11.8)
137 (17.2)	84 (8.0)	280 (10.9)
660 (82.8)	970 (92.0)	2,276 (89.1)

10

Adapted from Akerblom JL[5]

Table 10-2: Relationship Between Quartiles of Total Cholesterol and Hazard Ratios in the Three Ethnic Groups of the North Manhattan Study

| | Caucasian | |
Quartile	Range (mg/dL)	HR (95% CI)
1	≥176.5	2.2 (1.2–4.1)[a]
2	176.6–200.0	1.7 (0.9–3.3)
3	200.1–228.5	1.4 (0.7–2.8)
4	>228.5	1.0

Cox proportional hazards model with time to death as the time variable: 95% confidence interval.

[a]P-value <0.05. The baseline quartile, quartile 4, includes individuals in the 75th-100th percentile.

[b]HR (hazard ratio) adjusted for age, sex, education, study cohort, body mass index, apolipoprotein E genotype, heart disease, hypertension, diabetes, stroke, dementia, and smoking status.

Furthermore, this survival bias might be more pronounced for African-American and Hispanic participants. In the US, among those born in 1900, whites had an estimated life expectancy of 47.6 years, while nonwhites had an estimated life expectancy of 33.0 years. Among individuals born in 1921, whites had an estimated life expectancy of 61.8 years, while nonwhites had an estimated life expectancy of 51.5 years.[7] Some of this earlier mortality may have been related to lipid-related conditions. However, the effect of cholesterol on mortality was similar among whites and African Americans, after adjustment for demographic factors and comor-

African American		Hispanic	
Range (mg/dL)	HR (95% CI)	Range (mg/dL)	HR (95% CI)
≤174.0	1.9 (1.2–3.0)[b]	≤171.0	0.8 (0.5–1.4)
174.1–198.0	1.2 (0.8–1.9)	171.1–196.0	0.8 (0.5–1.3)
198.1–227.5	1.0 (0.6–1.6)	196.1–223.0	0.7 (0.4–1.2)
>227.5	1.0	>223.0	1.0

Only total cholesterol is shown. Similar trends were shown with LDL.

CI=confidence interval

Adapted from Akerblom JL[5]

bid conditions. This observation contrasted the findings in Hispanics, which suggest that healthy survival bias among nonwhites cannot entirely account for the observed results.

Aronow[8] reported the prevalence and incidence of cardiovascular disease (CVD) in older men and women in a long-term health-care facility. The cohort consisted of 1,160 men, mean age 80 +/- 8 years, and 2,464 women, mean age 81 +/- 8 years, and the mean follow-up was 46 +/- 30 months. The prevalence of hypertension, pacemaker rhythm, coronary artery disease (CAD), and thromboembolic stroke was similar in men and women. The prevalence of atrial fibrillation (AF) was higher in men (16%) than in women (13%; $P=0.019$), as was the prevalence of peripheral arterial disease (PAD) in men (32%) and women (26%; $P=0.0001$). At the 46-month follow-up, the incidences of new coronary events, thromboembolic stroke, and coronary heart failure (CHF) were similar in men and women.

The relationship between serum lipids and mortality in the elderly creates an interesting therapeutic dilemma for physicians. The National Cholesterol Education Program Adult Treatment Panel III (NCEP ATP III) guidelines[9] promoted the need to treat elderly people aggressively because the impact of total serum cholesterol on risk of CHD increases with age. Most men in their 70s carry a 10-year global risk of 12% by virtue of their age alone, which would place them in the intermediate risk category (see Figure 3-1, Chapter 3). Total serum cholesterol of 200 mg/dL would also place such men in the second quartile of risk (Table 10-2), and thus an attempt to lower it further could increase their risk of death.

A great deal of debate involves the safety and efficacy of lipid-lowering therapy in older patients and, although the risk of myopathy increases with age, the consensus is that these lipid-lowering drugs are safe in this segment of the population.[10] Of greater concern is the efficacy of these drugs as primary prevention for otherwise healthy elderly people. Ali et al[11] have reviewed the evidence in this regard. Their review was based on an extensive perusal of the literature and yielded six publications, which addressed the use of statins for primary prevention, three of which included subjects >75 years of age. Their conclusion contained a tepid endorsement that "the existing evidence suggests, but does not confirm, benefit from the use of statins for primary prevention in the elderly subgroup (ie, those aged >65 yr)."[11]

Hypertension

Several clinical trials have established the efficacy of blood pressure-lowering medications in reducing cardiovascular events. The age-specific effects of treatment were established by a collaborative meta-analysis from 61 prospective observational studies.[12] During 12.7 million person-years at risk, 56,000 vascular deaths (12,000 stroke, 34,000 ischemic heart disease [IHD], 10,000 other vascular), and 66,000 other deaths occurred in patients 40 to 89 years of age. Up to the time of death, there is a linear relationship between the risk of death from a cardiovascular cause and both systolic blood pressure (SBP) and diastolic blood pressure (DBP) (Figure 10-2). This relationship is depicted in a series of regression lines whose elevation increases with age. Each line extends down to a lower limit of SBP and DBP of 115 mm Hg and 75 mm Hg, respectively. At 40 to 69 years of age, each difference of 20 mm Hg in usual SBP or 10 mm Hg in usual DBP is associated with more than a twofold difference in the stroke death rate, and with twofold differences in the death rates from IHD and from other vascular causes. All of these proportional differences in vascular mortality are about half as extreme at 40 to 49 years of age as at 80 to 89 years of age, but the annual absolute differences in risk are greater in old age (Figure 10-2). The age-specific associations are similar for men and women, and for cerebral hemorrhage and cerebral ischemia. It was found that for predicting vascular mortality from a single blood pressure measurement, the average of SBP and DBP was slightly more informative than either alone, and pulse pressure was much less informative.[12]

While the effect of treatment is not a matter for debate, the discussion continues about the most effective therapy for individuals in the older age group, and some guidelines recommend the selective use of particular drug regimens based on patients' age.[14] This might reflect true comparability of the effects of reducing blood pressure in people of different age groups, but it could also be a function of the paucity of participants in the older age groups in clinical trials. This issue was addressed in a second meta-analysis undertaken with the intention of quantifying the relative risk reductions achieved with different regimens to lower blood pressure

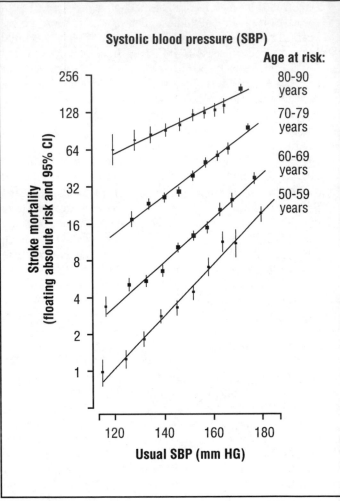

Figure 10-2: Stroke mortality rate in each decade of age versus usual blood pressure at the start of that decade. Rates are plotted on a floating absolute scale, and each square has area inversely proportional to the effective variance of the log mortality rate. For diastolic blood pressure, each age-specific

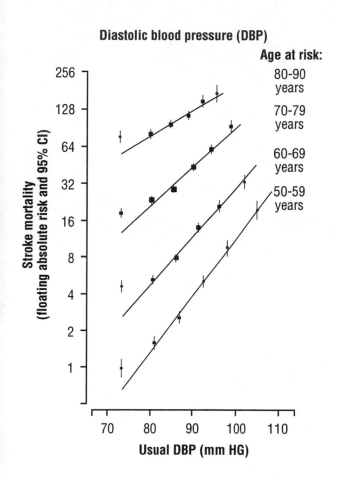

Diastolic blood pressure (DBP)

Age at risk:
80-90 years
70-79 years
60-69 years
50-59 years

Stroke mortality (floating absolute risk and 95% CI)

Usual DBP (mm HG)

regression line ignores the left-hand point (ie, at slightly less than 75 mm Hg), for which the risk lies significantly above the fitted regression line (as indicated by the broken line below 75 mm Hg). Used with permission from Lewington S, et al.[12] Note: the scale on the ordinate is a geometric progression.

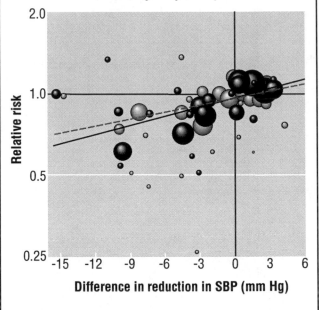

Figure 10-3: Associations of reduction in blood pressure with risk reduction for total major cardiovascular events for adults <65 and ≥65 years of age. Area of each circle is proportional to inverse variance of log odds ratio. Fitted lines represent summary meta-regressions for total major cardiovascular events. Used with permission from the Blood Pressure Lowering Treatment Trialists' Collaboration.[13]

in younger and older adults (<65 vs ≥65 yr). The analysis included 31 trials, with 190,606 participants, and showed no clear difference between age groups in the effects of lowering blood pressure or any difference between the effects of the drug classes on major cardiovascular events (all $P ≥0.24$)[13] (Figure 10-3). No significant interaction occurred between age and treatment when age was fitted as a continuous variable (all $P >0.09$). The meta-regressions also showed no difference in effects between the two age groups for the outcome of major cardiovascular events (<65 vs ≥65; $P=0.38$). Investigators concluded that reduction of blood pressure produces benefits in younger (<65 yr) and older (≥65 yr) adults, with no strong evidence that protection against major vascular events afforded by different drug classes varies substantially with age (Figures 10-4 and 10-5).[13]

Isolated Systolic Hypertension

Systolic blood pressure increases with age at least until the eighth decade of life, while diastolic pressure rises only up to the fifth decade, when it levels off or even drops slightly (Figure 10-6). The prevalence of isolated systolic hypertension varies not only with age, but also with gender and race. It is higher in women and in black subjects compared to Caucasians.[15] Staessen et al performed a meta-analysis of studies that reported the outcomes in placebo-controlled studies for treatment of isolated systolic hypertension. All the patients were 60 years of age or more and had SBP ≥160 mm Hg and DBP <95 mm Hg. In eight trials, 15,693 patients with isolated systolic hypertension were followed up for 3.8 years (median). After correction for regression dilution bias, sex, age, and DBP, the relative hazard rates associated with a 10 mm Hg higher initial SBP were 1.26 ($P=0.0001$) for total mortality, 1.22 ($P=0.02$) for stroke, but only 1.07 ($P=0.37$) for coronary events. Independent of SBP, DBP was inversely correlated with total mortality, highlighting the role of pulse pressure as a risk factor. Active treatment reduced total mortality by 13% (95% CI 2-22, $P=0.02$),

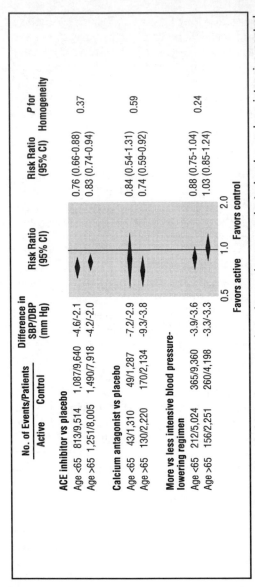

	No. of Events/Patients		Difference in SBP/DBP (mm Hg)	Risk Ratio (95% CI)	Risk Ratio (95% CI)	P for Homogeneity
	Active	Control				
ACE inhibitor vs placebo						
Age <65	813/9,514	1,087/9,640	-4.6/-2.1		0.76 (0.66-0.88)	0.37
Age >65	1,251/8,005	1,490/7,918	-4.2/-2.0		0.83 (0.74-0.94)	
Calcium antagonist vs placebo						
Age <65	43/1,310	49/1,287	-7.2/-2.9		0.84 (0.54-1.31)	0.59
Age >65	130/2,220	170/2,134	-9.3/-3.8		0.74 (0.59-0.92)	
More vs less intensive blood pressure-lowering regimen						
Age <65	212/5,024	365/9,360	-3.9/-3.6		0.88 (0.75-1.04)	0.24
Age >65	156/2,251	260/4,198	-3.3/-3.3		1.03 (0.85-1.24)	

0.5   1.0   2.0

Favors active   Favors control

Figure 10-4: Comparison of blood pressure-lowering regimens against placebo or less intensive control. SBP/DBP difference=overall difference in mean blood pressure during follow-up between treatment groups (actively treated group vs control group), calculated by weighting difference observed in each contributing trial by number of individuals in trial. Negative blood pressure values indicate lower mean follow-up blood pressure in first listed than in second listed groups. Used with permission from the Blood Pressure Lowering Treatment Trialists' Collaboration.[13]

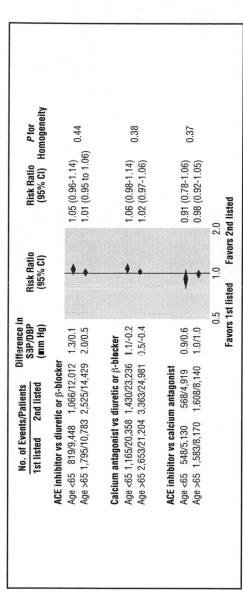

Figure 10-5: Blood pressure-lowering regimens based on different drug classes for the outcome of total major cardiovascular events and age groups <65 versus ≥65 years of age. Systolic blood pressure/diastolic blood pressure difference equals overall difference in mean blood pressure during follow-up between treatment groups (group assigned first listed treatment versus group assigned second listed treatment), calculated by weighting difference observed in each contributing trial by number of individuals in trial. Negative blood pressure values indicate lower mean follow-up blood pressure in first listed than in second listed groups. Used with permission from the Blood Pressure Lowering Treatment Trialists' Collaboration.[13]

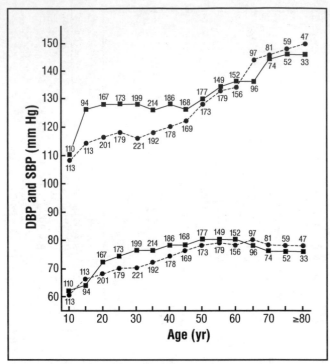

Figure 10-6: Systolic and diastolic blood pressures in 5-year age classes in a representative sample of the population of five Belgian districts. Each subject had the blood pressure measured five times on two separate home visits. The numbers in the diagram represent the number of subjects at each age range. ■ Males (n=2,044), ● Females (n= 2,158). Used with permission from Staessen J, et al.[15]

cardiovascular mortality by 18%, all cardiovascular complications by 26%, stroke by 30%, and coronary events by 23%. The number of patients to treat for 5 years to prevent one major cardiovascular event was lower in men (18 vs 38), at or above 70 years of age (19 vs 39), and in patients with previous cardiovascular complications (16 vs 37).

The authors suggested that drug treatment was justified in older patients with isolated systolic hypertension whose SBP was 160 mm Hg or higher. Absolute benefit is larger in men, in patients 70 years of age or more, and in those with previous cardiovascular complications or wider pulse pressure. Treatment prevented stroke more effectively than it did coronary events.[16] Similar benefits were also noted by several other trials not included in the meta-analysis.[17] These studies provide compelling evidence that isolated systolic hypertension should be treated energetically with conventional regimens of therapy.

Heart Failure

Heart failure is recognized as one of the main causes for hospitalization in people over 65 years of age. Nearly 5 million people are believed to have the disease in the US, and concerns mount about the potential burden this will impose on the health-care system in the US in the next few decades. Much of this discussion stems from reports based on hospital records, such as in the study reported by Fang et al.[18] They examined the National Hospital Discharge Survey data from 1979 to 2004 and assessed trends in hospitalizations for heart failure as either a first-listed or additional (second to seventh) diagnosis. They found that the number of hospitalizations with any mention of heart failure tripled, from 1.27 million in 1979 to 3.86 million in 2004; 65% to 70% of admissions were patients with additional diagnoses of heart failure. Heart failure hospitalization rates increased sharply with age. More than 80% of hospitalizations were among patients of at least 65 years of age and were paid by Medicare/Medicaid.

While findings of this nature are alarming, recent studies using more accurate diagnostic criteria cast some doubt about the authenticity of this epidemic of heart failure. The study conducted among the population of Olmsted County, Minnesota (the characteristics of which are similar to those of US, non-Hispanic whites), sought to address these con-

10

cerns because the Mayo Clinic and Olmsted Medical Center provide the majority of medical care for this population and also use a common system of medical records and coding illnesses.[19] Critical to this assessment were codes used for diagnosing heart failure, which were as follows: 428 (heart failure), 402.01 (hypertensive heart disease malignant with congestive heart failure), 402.11 (hypertensive heart disease benign with congestive heart failure), 425 (cardiomyopathy), 429.3 (cardiomegaly), and 514 (pulmonary congestion). Codes 402.91 (hypertensive heart disease unspecified with congestive heart failure), 404.01 (malignant hypertensive heart and renal disease with heart failure), 404.11 (benign hypertensive heart and renal disease with congestive heart failure), and 404.91 (unspecified hypertensive heart and renal disease with congestive heart failure) were queried, but not used as part of the coding practices during the study.

The incidence of heart failure was higher among men (378/100,000 persons for men; 289/100,000 persons for women) and did not change over time among men or women. Survival after heart failure diagnosis was worse among men than women (RR, 1.33) but overall survival improved over time (5-year, age-adjusted survival, 43% in 1979-1984 vs 52% in 1996-2000, $P <0.001$). However, men and young individuals experienced larger survival gains, contrasting with less or no improvement for women and elderly persons. This study highlighted another important facet of the heart failure "epidemic" in that nearly a third of the patients with heart failure were diagnosed in the outpatient setting and would not ordinarily appear as hospital admissions. For unknown reasons, the incidence of heart failure in this population was somewhat higher than that reported from the Framingham Heart Study (see National Institutes of Health [NIH] report). Nevertheless, the important aspect of the study reported by Roger et al[19] was that the incidence of heart failure was unchanged for the 20 years preceding 2000.

The age-adjusted, 5-year mortality estimates declined over time, with an overall improvement from 57% in 1979 to

1984 to 48% from 1996 to 2000 (P <0.01). However, there were age and sex differences in the degree of improvement in survival (P <0.001 for year-by-age interaction and year-by-sex interaction). Men in their 60s experienced a 52% improvement in survival between corresponding periods. Survival also improved, although to a lesser degree, among older men. Among women, survival improved in younger ages, but to a lesser extent than it did among men, and it did not change in older age groups (Table 10-3).[19]

The essential nature of the epidemic of heart failure was addressed in a more recent report by Curtis et al.[20] This study was possibly the largest one that addressed the incidence and prevalence of heart failure in those >65 years of age. The authors analyzed medical records of a 5% sample of Medicare beneficiaries and the corresponding denominator files from 1994 to 2003. The analysis included both inpatient and outpatient records, and focused on a selection of International Classification of Diseases (ICD)-9 CM codes, which provided >95% specificity for a diagnosis of heart failure. The overall prevalence and incidence of heart failure were slightly higher than those observed in the study by Roger et al.[19] The incidence of heart failure declined from 32 per 1,000 person-years in 1994 to 29 per 1,000 person-years in 2003 (P <0.01). Incidence declined most sharply among beneficiaries 80 to 84 years of age (from 57.5 to 48.4 per 1,000 person-years, P <0.01) and increased slightly among beneficiaries aged 65 to 69 years (from 17.5 to 19.3 per 1,000 person-years, P <0.01). As expected, the incidence was significantly greater in older Medicare beneficiaries (Figure 10-7). The prevalence increased from ~90/1,000 Medicare beneficiaries in 1994 to ~121/1,000 in 2003.

In terms of overall survival, modest reductions in mortality occurred at 30 days, 1 year, and 5 years. The median survival after the incident diagnosis was 2.9 years, with a slightly better outlook for women (3.1 yr vs 2.7 yr). Although risk-adjusted mortality declined slightly from 1994 to 2003, the prognosis for patients diagnosed with heart failure re-

Table 10-3: Relative Risk of Death After the Initial Diagnosis of Heart Failure in Men and Women Relative to Age

Relative Risk (95% CI)

Men

Age, yr	1979-1984	1985-1990
60	1.00	0.84 (0.69-1.02)
70	1.00	0.84 (0.73-0.97)
80	1.00	0.85 (0.72-1.00)

Women

Age, yr	1979-1984	1985-1990
60	1.00	0.80 (0.63-1.03)
70	1.00	0.91 (0.77-1.06)
80	1.00	1.02 (0.90-1.15)

CI=confidence interval
Used with permission from Roger VL, et al[19]

mained poor. In 2002, risk-adjusted, 1-year mortality was 27.5%, more than three times higher than for age- and sex-matched patients (Figure 10-8).

Comorbidities in the Elderly With Heart Failure

Elderly patients with heart failure often have comorbidities. This factor will likely influence the long-term outlook in these patients, even though multiple clinical trials during the last two decades have identified therapies that are

1991-1995	1996-2000
0.63 (0.50-0.80)	0.48 (0.36-0.64)
0.74 (0.63-0.88)	0.59 (0.49-0.71)
0.88 (0.75-1.04)	0.72 (0.61-0.87)

1991-1995	1996-2000
0.95 (0.73-1.24)	0.67 (0.48-0.92)
0.99 (0.83-1.18)	0.79 (0.64-0.98)
1.03 (0.90-1.17)	0.94 (0.82-1.09)

effective in managing people with chronic heart failure. Little is known about whether or not the improvements are reflected in trends in early and long-term mortality and hospital readmissions for heart failure (see Chapter 7). A retrospective cohort study of 2.5 million elderly Medicare beneficiaries hospitalized with heart failure between January 1, 2001, and December 31, 2005, provided some interesting insights.[21] Unadjusted in-hospital mortality declined from 5.1% to 4.2% during the study ($P <0.001$),

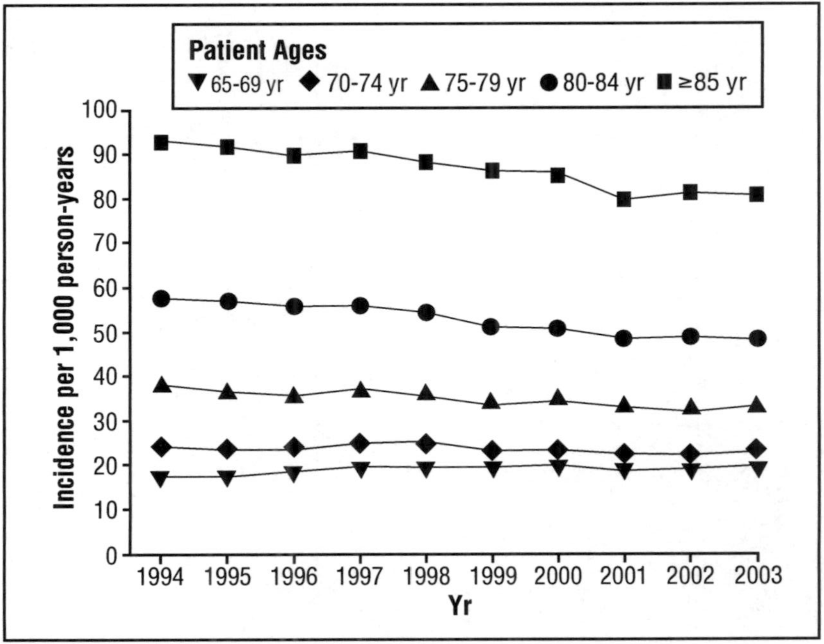

Figure 10-7: Age-specific incidence of heart failure among Medicare beneficiaries from January 1, 1994, through December 31, 2003. The incidence of heart failure increased slightly among the youngest Medicare beneficiaries and declined among older beneficiaries. Used with permission from Curtis LH.[20]

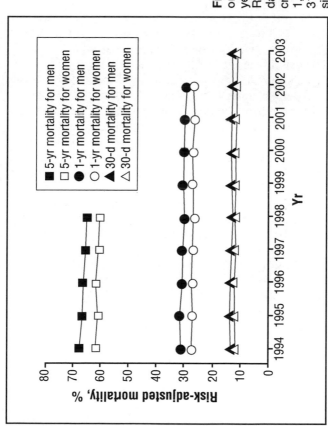

Figure 10-8: Mortality after onset of heart failure by year of incidence and sex. Risk-adjusted mortality at 30 days, 1 year, and 5 years decreased slightly from January 1, 1994, through December 31, 2003. Used with permission from Curtis LH.[21]

but 30-day, 180-day, and 1-year all-cause mortality remained fairly constant at 11%, 26%, and 37%, respectively. Nearly 1 in 4 patients were readmitted within 30 days of the index hospitalization, and two-thirds were readmitted within 1 year. Controlling for patient- and hospital-level covariates, the hazard of all-cause mortality at 1 year was slightly lower in 2005 than in 2001 (hazard ratio [HR], 0.98; 95%: CI, 0.97-0.99). The hazard of readmission did not decline significantly from 2001 to 2005 (HR, 0.99; 95%: CI, 0.98-1.00).

More than 1 in 10 Medicare beneficiaries died, and more than 1 in 5 were readmitted to the hospital within 30 days of hospitalization for heart failure. Nearly half of the readmissions were for cardiovascular causes, a finding that is not surprising given the paucity of therapeutic options with demonstrated benefit for early outcomes.[22] In this regard, no placebo-controlled study has shown a short-term survival benefit or decreased hospitalizations following acute heart failure.

Long-term outcomes were similarly poor. During 1 year of follow-up, more than 1 in 3 Medicare beneficiaries died, and two-thirds were readmitted to the hospital. Nearly 40% of patients were admitted at least twice. At first glance, these findings may seem surprising, given the demonstrated survival benefit associated with treatment with angiotensin-converting enzyme (ACE) inhibitors and β-blockers in clinical trials of patients with heart failure. Several factors may explain the discrepancy. First, clinical trials often exclude elderly patients, and databases to examine the effectiveness of therapies for treating heart failure in elderly patients are limited. There is evidence, however, that patients who may benefit the most from treatment with β-blockers, ACE inhibitors, and angiotensin receptor blockers (ARBs) may be the least likely to receive them.[21,23,24]

Cardiovascular and respiratory diagnosis-related groups (DRGs) dominated readmissions, but renal failure and gastrointestinal (GI) hemorrhage were not uncommon. Only a quarter of readmissions were specifically for heart failure, 3% of readmissions were for renal failure, and 2.5% were for GI hemorrhage with comorbidity and complications. Readmission for ICD implantation rose steadily from 0.3% in 2001 to 1.2% in 2005.

Atrial Fibrillation

Atrial fibrillation (AF) is a common arrhythmia in elderly persons and an important cause of embolic stroke. While most studies of the prevalence of AF have used selected, hospital-based populations, the Cardiovascular Health Study (CHS) was a population-based, longitudinal study of risk factors for CAD and stroke in 5,201 men and women, ≥65 years of age. Atrial fibrillation was diagnosed in 4.8% of women and in 6.2% of men at the baseline examination, and prevalence was strongly associated with advanced age in women.[25] Admissions to hospital for this condition as a primary diagnosis have been increasing steadily over the last two decades. Hospitalizations for AF are approximately eight times more in people over 65 years of age compared to those less than 65 years of age (Figure 10-9).[26] Management of this condition rests on a choice between rate control with medications or cardioversion to restore sinus rhythm, both being undertaken against a background of adequate anticoagulation to prevent strokes.

The average yearly risk of stroke is 5%, and this risk is increased in the presence of certain factors, including left ventricular (LV) dysfunction, hypertension, history of stroke, diabetes, heart failure, and increasing age. Long-term antithrombotic therapy with warfarin or aspirin reduces of the risk of a stroke in these patients by 68% and 21%, respectively. There is no convincing evidence that these RR reductions vary according to patients' baseline chance of stroke. Therefore, among all age groups, elderly persons would receive the greatest absolute benefit from warfarin or aspirin prophylaxis. However, one consideration that arises in dealing with elderly individuals is the

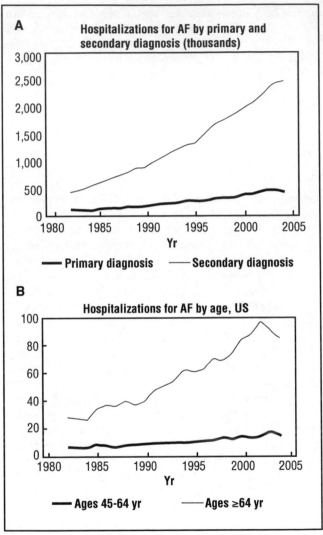

Figure 10-9A and B: Hospitalizations for atrial fibrillation (AF). A: Total; B: Admission by age. From the National Institutes of Health Chartbook.[26]

risk of falls. A Markov decision-analytic model has been used to determine the preferred treatment strategy (no antithrombotic therapy, long-term aspirin use, or long-term warfarin use) for patients with AF who are 65 years of age and older and are at risk for falling, and have no other contraindications to antithrombotic therapy. Input data were obtained by systematic review of Medline, and outcomes were expressed as quality-adjusted life-years. For patients with average risks of stroke and falling, warfarin therapy was associated with 12.90 quality-adjusted life-years per patient; aspirin therapy, 11.17 quality-adjusted life-years; and no antithrombotic therapy, 10.15 quality-adjusted life-years. Sensitivity analysis demonstrated that, regardless of the patient's age or baseline risk of stroke, the risk of falling was not an important factor in determining their optimal antithrombotic therapy.[27] In elderly people with AF and no additional comorbidities, there is evidence that AF is a marker for other cardiovascular events and should be viewed as an indication for anticoagulation.[28]

Aortic Stenosis

Aortic valve sclerosis is the calcification and thickening of a trileaflet aortic valve in the absence of obstruction to ventricular outflow.[29] It is a forerunner of frank aortic stenosis, which causes obstruction to LV outflow, left ventricular hypertrophy (LVH), and ultimately heart failure, ischemia, and/or syncope. The frequency of aortic stenosis increases with age, making it a major geriatric problem in people >65 years of age. The incidence of aortic stenosis increases with age, male gender, smoking, hypertension, high lipoprotein(a), high LDL, and diabetes mellitus. Aortic valves affected by aortic stenosis contain a higher amount of oxidized LDL cholesterol (LDL-C) and show increased expression of metalloproteinases. Aortic stenosis can be suspected in the presence of an ejection systolic murmur at the aortic area, decreased intensity of the second heart sound, and slow carotid upstroke; but it can be best detected by echocardiography. Aortic stenosis may be accompanied by mitral annulus calcification in nearly 50% of cases. It is associated with an increase of approximately 50% in the risk of death from cardiovascular causes and the risk of myocardial infarction (MI).

It has been reported recently that age alone is often used as a criterion to deny surgical treatment in these patients.[30] The results of surgical therapy have been remarkable even in octogenarians. A retrospective analysis of 277 individuals ≥80 years of age who had a diagnosis of severe aortic stenosis (aortic valve [AV] area ≤0.8 cm^2) between 1993 and 2003 was performed to determine long-term outcomes.[31] Survival curves of patients who underwent aortic valve replacement (AVR) during the follow-up period were compared with those managed nonsurgically. The patients in the first group had an average age of 85+/-4 years (53% male) and an aortic valve area of 0.68+/-0.16 cm^2 (normal = 3-4 cm^2). The ejection fraction (EF) was 52+/-20%, 47% had CHD, and 17% had diabetes. Over a mean follow-up of 2.5 years, 55 (20%) had AVR, and there were a total of 175 deaths.

One-year, 2-year, and 5-year survival rates among patients with AVR were 87%, 78%, and 68%, respectively, compared with 52%, 40%, and 22%, respectively, in those who had no AVR (P <0.0001). Hazard ratio for death with AVR adjusted for 19 covariates, including age, EF, gender, comorbidities, and pharmacotherapy, was 0.38 (95% CI 0.26-0.66, P <0.0001). The analysis concluded that the prognosis of medically managed, severe, calcific aortic stenosis in the elderly patients is poor, surgical treatment appears to improve survival of these patients, and surgical treatment should be strongly considered in the absence of other major comorbidities. A similar retrospective analysis was undertaken in octogenarian patients who had undergone aortic valve surgery in Milan. The overall 5-year survival was similar to Pai et al.[31] The latter also observed a slightly better outcome in those who had a mechanical valve compared to those with a biological prosthesis.[32]

Summary

In terms of managing risk factors for CHD, treatment of hypertension ranks as the least problematic. The evidence suggests that hyperlipidemia should also be treated despite the inverse relationship between total cholesterol and mortality. Atrial fibrillation should be treated in the same way that it is with younger people and should include an effective embolic stroke-prevention regimen. Aortic stenosis should be managed in a manner similar to that in younger patients.

References

1.   Centers for Disease Control and Prevention: The state of aging and health in America 2007. www.cdc.gov/Aging/pdf/saha_2007.pdf. Accessed July 7, 2009.

2.   Wan H, Sengupta M, Velkoff VA, et al: US Census Bureau: 65+ in the United States: 2005. 2005:23-209.

3.   Centers for Disease Control and Prevention: Trends in causes of death among older persons in the United States. www.cdc. gov/nchs/data/ahcd/agingtrends/06olderpersons.pdf. Accessed June 22, 2009.

4.   White AD, Hames CG, Tyroler HA: Serum cholesterol and 20-year mortality in black and white men and women aged 65 and older in the Evans County Heart Study. *Ann Epidemiol* 1992;2:85-91.

5.   Akerblom JL, Costa R, Luchsinger JA, et al: Relation of plasma lipids to all-cause mortality in Caucasian, African-American and Hispanic elders. *Age Ageing* 2008; 37:207-213.

6.   Schupf N, Costa R, Luchsinger J, et al: Relationship between plasma lipids and all-cause mortality in nondemented elderly. *J Am Geriatr Soc* 2005;53:219-226.

7.   National Vital Statistics Reports: 2004;53:33-34. www.cdc. gov/nchs/data/nvsr/nvsr53/nvsr53_06.pdf. Accessed June 29, 2009.

8.   Aronow WS, Ahn C, Gutstein H: Prevalence and incidence of cardiovascular disease in 1160 older men and 2464 older women in a long-term health care facility. *J Gerontol A Biol Sci Med Sci* 2002;57: M45-46.

9.   Expert Panel on Detection, Evaluation, and Treatment of High Blood Cholesterol in Adults: Executive summary of the Third Report

of the National Cholesterol Education Program (NCEP) Expert Panel on Detection, Evaluation and Treatment of High Blood Cholesterol in Adults (Adult Treatment Panel III). *JAMA* 2001;285:2486-2497.

10. Jacobson TA: Overcoming the ageism bias in the treatment of hypercholesterolemia—A review of safety of statins in the elderly. *Drug Safety* 2006;29:421-445.

11. Ali R, Alexander KP: Statins for the primary prevention of cardiovascular events in older adults: a review of the evidence. *Am J Geriatr Pharmacother* 2007;5:52-63.

12. Lewington S, Clarke R, Qizilbash N, et al: Prospective Studies Collaboration. Age-specific relevance of usual blood pressure to vascular mortality: a meta-analysis of individual data for one million adults in 61 prospective studies. *Lancet* 2002;360(9349):1903-1913.

13. Blood Pressure Lowering Treatment Trialists' Collaboration: Effects of different regimens to lower blood pressure on major cardiovascular events in older and younger adults: meta-analysis of randomised trials. *BMJ* 2008;336:1121-1123.

14. Khan NA, Hemmelgarn B, Padwal R, et al: Canadian Hypertension Education Program. The 2007 Canadian Hypertension Education Program recommendations for the management of hypertension: part 2 - Therapy. *Can J Cardiol* 2007;23:539-550.

15. Staessen J, Amery A, Fagard R: Isolated systolic hypertension in the elderly. *J Hypertens* 1990;8:393-405.

16. Staessen JA, Gasowski J, Wang JG, et al: Risks of untreated and treated isolated systolic hypertension in the elderly: meta-analysis of outcome trials. *Lancet* 2000;355(9207):865-872.

17. Insua JT, Sacks HS, Lau TS, et al: Drug treatment of hypertension in the elderly: a meta-analysis. *Ann Intern Med* 1994;121:355-362.

18. Fang J, Mensah GA, Croft JB, et al: Heart failure-related hospitalization in the U.S., 1979 to 2004. *J Am Coll Cardiol* 2008;52: 428-434.

19. Roger VL, Weston SA, Redfield MM, et al: Trends in heart failure incidence and survival in a community-based population *JAMA* 2004;292:344-350.

20. Curtis LH, Greiner MA, Hammill BG, et al: Incidence and prevalence of heart failure in elderly persons, 1994-2003. *Arch Intern Med* 2008;168:418-424.

21. Curtis LH, Whellan DJ, Hammill BG, et al: Early and long-term outcomes of heart failure in elderly persons, 2001-2005. *Arch Intern Med* 2008;168:2481-2488.

22. Lloyd-Jones DM, Larson ML, Leip EP, et al: Lifetime risk for developing congestive heart failure: the Framingham Heart Study. *Circulation* 2002;106:3068-3072.

23. Lee DS, Tu JV, Juurlink DN, et al: Risk-treatment mismatch in the pharmacotherapy of heart failure. *JAMA* 2005;294:1240-1247.

24. Smith N, Chan J, Rea T, et al: Time trends in the use of β-blockers and other pharmacotherapies in older adults with congestive heart failure. *Am Heart J* 2004;148:710-717.

25. Furberg CD, Psaty MB, Manolio TA, et al: Prevalence of atrial fibrillation in elderly subjects (the cardiovascular health study) *Am J Cardiol* 1994;74:236-241.

26. National Institutes of Health Chart Book: www.nhlbi.nih.gov/resources/docs/07-chtbk.pdf. Accessed June 29, 2009.

27. Man-Son-Hing M, Nichol, G, Lau A, et al: Choosing antithrombotic therapy for elderly patients with atrial fibrillation who are at risk for falls. *Arch Intern Med* 1999;159:677-685.

28. Kopecky SL, Gersh BJ, McGoon MD, et al: Lone atrial fibrillation in elderly persons: a marker for cardiovascular risk. *Arch Intern Med* 1999;159:1118-1122.

29. Prasad Y, Bhalodkar NC: Aortic sclerosis—a marker of coronary atherosclerosis. *Clin Cardiol* 2004;27:671-673.

30. Bramstedt KA: Aortic valve replacement in the elderly: frequently indicated yet frequently denied. *Gerontology* 2003;49:46-49.

31. Pai RG, Varadarajan P, Kapoor N, et al: Aortic valve replacement improves survival in severe aortic stenosis associated with severe pulmonary hypertension. *Ann Thorac Surg* 2007;84:80-85.

32. de Vincentiis C, Kunkl AB, Trimarchi S, et al: Aortic valve replacement in octogenarians: is biologic valve the unique solution? *Ann Thorac Surg* 2008;85:1296-1301.

10

Chapter 11

Cardiovascular Disease in Children

By Laura L. Hayman, PhD, RN

ardiovascular disease (CVD) remains a major cause of premature mortality and morbidity in women and men in the United States and in most countries.[1] Atherosclerotic CVD begins early in childhood and develops over the life course by the interaction of genetic factors, potentially modifiable behaviors, and environmental exposures. During the past four decades, evidence from clinical studies has contributed to our understanding of the origins and progression of CVD processes. These data provide convincing support for beginning CVD prevention early in life. This chapter provides an overview of this evidence and reviews current guidelines and recommendations for prevention efforts to optimize cardiovascular health for children and youth and reduce the risk and burden of CVD in adult life.

The Evidence for CVD Prevention in Childhood

While no data from randomized, controlled trials (RCTs) demonstrate that risk reduction interventions in childhood prevent CVD in adult life, much of the evidence argues convincingly for CVD prevention beginning early in life. Autopsy data from the Bogalusa Heart Study (BHS) and the Pathobiological Determinants of Atherosclerosis in Youth (PDAY) study confirmed the importance of potentially modifiable risk factors and behaviors, including atherogenic lipids (non-high-density lipoprotein cholesterol [non-HDL-C]), HDL-cholesterol (HDL-C), hypertension, tobacco use, and obesity.[2-4] Specifically, autopsy data from BHS indicate the presence of reversible lesions (fatty streaks) in the aorta by 10 years of age and in the coronary arteries by the second decade of life.[2,3] Reports from PDAY, similar to observations made during the Korean War, confirmed the presence of atherosclerotic plaques in approximately 15% of individuals by 20 years of age.[4-8] Particularly noteworthy observations in BHS and PDAY link modifiable risk factors and behaviors with the extent of lesions in the aorta and coronary arteries.[2-4] The most extensive plaque involvement was observed in individuals who had multiple risk factors in early life.[2-4]

Noninvasive imaging has also been used to examine the association of potentially modifiable risk factors for CVD with vascular structure and function in childhood and adolescence and atherosclerosis in young adult life. A report from the Muscatine Study, a longitudinal, observational study of CVD risk factors in children and youth, used carotid ultrasound in adults 33 to 42 years of age and found that carotid intima-media thickness (CIMT) was positively associated with levels of total serum cholesterol and body mass index (BMI) measured in childhood.[9] Results from the BHS were similar: childhood levels of low-density lipoprotein cholesterol (LDL-C) and BMI predicted increased CIMT in adulthood.[10]

Finally, data from the Young Finns Study, a population-based prospective cohort study of 2,229 young adults 24 to 39 years of age, link risk factor exposures in 12- to 18-year-olds and CIMT in adult life.[11] The potentially modifiable risk factors and behaviors that predicted preclinical atherosclerosis included LDL-C, BMI, cigarette smoking, and systolic blood pressure (SBP).[11]

These data were bolstered by data on the tracking of risk factors from childhood to young adulthood,[12-14] by epidemiologic data on the prevalence of risk factors and adverse health behaviors,[1,15-16] and by more limited data on the safety and efficacy of modifying risk factors and adverse health behaviors in childhood and adolescence.[1,17,18] Taken together, these data prompted scientific guidelines for cardiovascular health promotion and risk reduction beginning early in life. For children and youth, healthy lifestyle behaviors and therapeutic lifestyle changes (TLC) are central to cardiovascular health promotion and risk reduction.

CVD Prevention Guidelines for Children and Youth

In 1992, the National Cholesterol Education Program (NCEP) Expert Panel on Blood Cholesterol Levels in Childhood issued the first set of guidelines for the assessment, evaluation, and treatment of dyslipidemias as part of CVD prevention in children and youth.[19] NCEP recommended a prudent diet, low in saturated fat and cholesterol (referred to as Step 1), for all healthy children 2 years of age and older with sufficient caloric intake to maintain growth and developmental processes. Based on available evidence, NCEP recommended an algorithm for screening, evaluation, and treatment of lipid disorders that focused on LDL-C levels. Selective, targeted screening for lipid disorders was recommended for at-risk children and adolescents if one of the following conditions were present:

(a) family history of myocardial infarction, angina pectoris, peripheral or cerebral vascular disease, or sudden death prior to age 55;

(b) parents and/or grandparents who required coronary artery bypass surgery or balloon angioplasty prior to age 55;

(c) parents with elevated total cholesterol (TC) levels (>240 mg/dL);

(d) unknown parent/grandparent family history *or* the child has two or more risk factors for coronary artery disease (CAD), including obesity (BMI >95th percentile for age and sex), hypertension, cigarette smoking, low HDL-C, physical inactivity/sedentary lifestyle, and diabetes mellitus.

For children and adolescents screened and identified with elevated levels of LDL-C, (borderline high: 110 mg/dL to 129 mg/dL; high: ≥130 mg/dL), the NCEP guidelines recommended an adequate trial (6 to 12 months) of TLC, including reduction of dietary saturated fat and cholesterol (referred to as Step II diet), increased physical activity, and normalization of body weight. The NCEP recommended drug therapy for children 10 years of age and older whose LDL-C levels remained ≥190 mg/dL. Concomitantly, diet therapy and TLC were recommended to enhance the treatment regimen.

Furthermore, the recommendations suggested that drug therapy should be considered in children whose LDL-C levels remained at ≥160 mg/dL and who have a family history of premature CVD (before 55 years of age) or two or more other CVD risk factors after vigorous attempts have been made to control these risk factors.[19]

When the recommendations were made in the early 1990s, bile acid sequestrants were the recommended drug of choice and HMG-CoA reductase inhibitors (statins) were not recommended for use in children. Since then, several studies of adolescents with genetic/familial dyslipidemias have demonstrated the safety and efficacy of statins in lowering LDL-C in children and adolescents.[20,21] A recent meta-analysis has reaffirmed these results.[22]

Based on accumulated data, the American Heart Association (AHA) issued a scientific statement in 2007 on drug therapy of high-risk lipid abnormalities in children and adolescents that modified the NCEP recommendations.[23] Those modifications include:

(a) in addition to family history, overweight and obesity should prompt screening with a fasting lipid profile;

(b) overweight and obese children with lipid abnormalities should be screened for other aspects of the metabolic syndrome (ie, insulin resistance and type 2 diabetes, hypertension, or central adiposity);

(c) for children meeting criteria for starting lipid-lowering drug therapy, a statin is recommended as first-line treatment;

(d) for children with high-risk lipid abnormalities, the presence of additional risk factors or high-risk conditions may lower the recommended cut point LDL-C level for initiation of drug therapy, lower the desired target LDL-C level, and, in selected cases, prompt consideration for initiation of treatment below 10 years of age. These risk factors and high-risk conditions may include male gender; strong family history of premature CVD or events; low HDL-C, high triglycerides (Tg), or small, dense lipoproteins; overweight or obesity and aspects of the metabolic syndrome; presence of other metabolic conditions associated with increased atherosclerotic risk, such as diabetes, HIV infection, systemic lupus erythematosus, organ transplantation, or survivor of childhood cancer; hypertension; current smoking and passive smoking exposure; and the presence of novel and emerging risk factors and markers, such as elevated lipoprotein(a), homocysteine, and C-reactive protein (CRP).[23]

The AHA statement also endorsed the need for ongoing research on drug therapy of high-risk lipid abnormalities in children, particularly the need for long-term safety and efficacy data and the impact on the atherosclerotic process.[23]

In 2008, the American Academy of Pediatrics (AAP) issued a statement on lipid screening and cardiovascular health in childhood[24] that was designed to reflect the evidence accrued since 1998, when the previous AAP report was published.[25] Prompted in part by the epidemic of childhood obesity and its comorbidities—including dyslipidemia, hypertension, and type 2 diabetes—the AAP statement emphasizes the need for CVD prevention in children and youth, the importance of adopting health-related lifestyle behaviors conducive to CV health, and the need to modify adverse patterns of dietary intake and physical inactivity.[24] Similar to the NCEP recommendations, the AAP 2008 statement supports a targeted approach to screening at-risk children, especially overweight and obese children, regardless of family history or other risk factors. The AAP 2008 recommendations are generally consistent with those issued by the AHA regarding identification and treatment of high-risk lipid abnormalities in children and youth[23] and with AHA guidelines for primary prevention of CVD.[26,27] Since these AAP recommendations[24] are the most current, their important points of emphasis are:

(a) a healthy diet in accordance with the US Department of Agriculture Center for Nutrition Policy and Promotion's Dietary Guidelines for Americans[28] should be recommended to all children older than 2 years of age, including the use of low-fat dairy products. For example, reduced-fat milk is considered appropriate for children between 12 months and 2 years of age for whom overweight is a concern or who have a family history of obesity, dyslipidemia, or CVD;

(b) for children and adolescents at higher risk for CVD and with elevated levels of LDL-C, dietary therapy with nutritional counseling and other TLC, including increased levels of physical activity, are recommended. Based on available safety and efficacy data, a diet low in saturated fat (<7% of daily calories) and dietary cholesterol (≤200 mg/day), supplemented with increasing intake of soluble fiber, is suggested. In addition, plant stanols and sterols, currently added to a number of food products, including spreads and margarines, orange juice, and cereal bars, lower the absorption of dietary cholesterol and have been shown to reduce cholesterol concentrations by 5% to 10% in adults with minimal adverse effects.[29] While minimal pediatric data exist, results of one RCT indicated that a margarine product resulting in 20 g/day intake of plant sterols reduced LDL-C by 8%.[30] Importantly, in terms of safety, plant sterols also result in decrease absorption of fat-soluble vitamins and betacarotene;

(c) selective, targeted screening of children and adolescents with a family history of dyslipidemia or premature CVD or dyslipidemia (≤55 years of age for men and ≤65 years of age for women) is supported. Similar to the AHA guidelines,[23] screening is also recommended for children and adolescents for whom family history is unknown or for those with other risk factors, including overweight, hypertension, cigarette smoking, sedentary lifestyle, or diabetes mellitus. Importantly, the AAP guidelines also recommend that a fasting lipid profile be obtained for children between 2 and 10 years of age and within the context of well-child care.

In view of the prevalence of childhood obesity and its association with multiple CVD risk factors, it seems prudent to recommend a baseline lipid screening and assessment in childhood (after age 2 when serum lipids begin to track and before the onset of puberty when hormonal and other physiologic changes affect lipid levels). Consistent with current recommendations,[24,31] this could optimally be done in the context of well-child care and maintained as part of the child's total CV and health profile.

While the safety and short-term efficacy of pharmacologic agents now recommended for treatment of dyslipidemia in children and adolescents have been established, controversy exists within the pediatric health-care community about the age of initiation of such therapies. We await the outcomes and recommendations of the National Heart, Lung and Blood Institute (NHLBI) Pediatric Risk Reduction Initiative to guide and inform clinical practice in this critically important area of child health;

(d) for overweight children and adolescents with high Tg concentrations or low cardioprotective HDL-C, weight management is recommended as primary treatment, including dietary therapy and counseling and increased physical activity as part of improving energy balance;

(e) pharmacologic interventions are recommended for consideration in children 8 years of age and older with

LDL-C levels ≥190 mg/dL (or ≥160 mg/dL with a family history of premature CVD, or ≥2 additional risk factors, or ≥130 mg/dL if diabetes mellitus is present). While the initial target goal is to lower LDL-C to <160 mg/dL, targets of 130 mg/dL or 110 mg/dL may be warranted, particularly in a child with a strong family history of CVD or with other risk factors.

The recent AAP recommendations provide an overview of pharmacotherapies now recommended for management of dyslipidemia in children and youth, including bile acid sequestrants, statins, and niacin; however, no recommendations for first-line medications are suggested.[24]

Health Behaviors as Central to Cardiovascular Health Promotion and Risk Reduction in Children and Adolescents

Health behaviors are a central component of primary prevention and cardiovascular risk reduction in children and youth. As previously discussed, an adequate trial of TLC with emphasis on normalization of body weight is recommended by AHA, AAP, and the NHLBI for initial management of most dyslipidemias and elevated blood pressure.[23,24,26,32,33] For cardiovascular risk reduction, many factors are considered before moving beyond TLC to pharmacotherapy, including the child's age and maturation level, total risk profile, family history of CVD, response to TLC, and patient and family preferences.[23,24,31] The Fourth Pediatric Report of the National High Blood Pressure Education Program provides guidelines for prevention and management of elevated blood pressure.[33] Similarly, the AAP Expert Panel report outlines a staged approach for prevention and management of overweight and obesity in children and youth.[32] Particularly noteworthy is the consensus across reports on the importance of health behaviors in managing cardiovascular risk factors in children and youth.

Health behaviors are the cornerstone of population-based as well as individual/clinical efforts focused on optimizing cardiovascular health and reducing the risk and burden of CVD across the life course. The AHA, the AAP, and other pediatric and public-health advocacy groups promote smoke-free lifestyles and environments, and healthy patterns of dietary intake and physical activity.[6,26,33-35] The AHA's most recent dietary recommendations for *all* children (≥2 years of age and older), endorsed by AAP and consistent with other public-health guidelines, emphasize a diet that relies on fruits and vegetables, whole grains, low-fat and nonfat dairy products, beans, fish, and lean meat.[35] With heart health as a major goal, the AHA continues to emphasize diets low in saturated fat, *trans* fat, and cholesterol and more liberal intakes of unsaturated fat, particularly ω-3 fatty acids.[35] Reducing sugars, sugar-sweetened beverages, and salt intake, including salt from processed foods, is emphasized in all recent dietary guidelines for children and youth.[28,35] A major point of emphasis in recent recommendations, prompted in part by the increase in prevalence of childhood obesity, is balancing dietary calories with physical activity to maintain normal growth and prevent overweight.[28,35] In addition, the Dietary Guidelines for Americans and the AHA now provide recommendations for essential and discretionary calories based on age, gender, and activity level, as well as specific guidelines for daily intakes of macronutrients and micronutrients.[28,35]

Reflecting accumulated evidence on the benefits of active lifestyles, current physical activity recommendations for healthy children and youth emphasize 60 min/day of moderate-to-vigorous physical activity (MVPA).[36] In addition, the US Department of Health & Human Services 2008 Physical Activity Guidelines for Americans call for vigorous activity and muscle and bone strengthening activities on at least three days per week.[37] Moderate level of intensity is 3.0 to 6.0 metabolic equivalents (METs), expending 3.5 to 7.0 kcal/min, while activity requiring greater than 6.0

METS is considered vigorous, expending more than 7.0 kcal/min. Similar to the recommendations for adults, the 60 min/day can be achieved through intermittent physical activity (ie, six 10-min sessions) and accumulated in a variety of settings.[37] A recent review of empirical literature on the associations between physical activity and health outcomes in children and youth provides evidence supporting these recommendations.[38] However, while the cardiovascular benefits of physically active lifestyles are well-documented, the degree of physical activity required to modify specific CVD risk factors in children and youth remains to be clarified.[38]

Schools and CVD Prevention in Children and Adolescents

Pediatric health-care providers and child-health advocacy groups understand that healthy diets, physical activity, and smoke-free lifestyles begin early in life and are influenced by numerous factors.[39,40] These factors include the child's family, school, and community. For example, the lack of required physical education in most US school systems today fails to promote physical activity in school-aged children and misses a critical opportunity for helping children meet the recommended guidelines of 60 min/day of MVPA. This is particularly true for children from racial and ethnic minority groups and low-income communities who are at risk for overweight. Similarly, the continued availability of nutrient-poor food in schools, such as the fare offered through vending machines, detracts from the gains made in federally-subsidized food programs and from the overall quality of school nutritional efforts. Schools are key venues for helping US children and youth to meet recommended goals for dietary intake and physical activity. Child-health professionals and child advocates have much work remaining to move these agendas forward on regional and national levels.[41,42]

References

1. American Heart Association: Heart Disease and Stroke Statistics: 2008 Update. Dallas, TX, 2008.

2. Newman WP III, Freedman DS, Coors AW, et al: Relation of serum lipoprotein levels and systolic blood pressure to early atherosclerosis. *N Engl J Med* 1986;314:138-144.

3. Berenson GS, Srinivasan SR, Bao W, et al for the Bogalusa Heart Study: Association between multiple cardiovascular risk factors and the early development of atherosclerosis. *N Engl J Med* 1998;338:1650-1656.

4. McGill HC, McMahan CA, Zieske AW, et al: Pathobiological Determinants of Atherosclerosis in Youth (PDAY) research group. Effect of nonlipid risk factors on atherosclerosis in youth with a favorable lipoprotein profile. *Circulation* 2001;103:1546-1555C.

5. Mahoney LT, Burns TL, Stanford W, et al: Coronary risk factors measured in childhood and young adult life are associated with coronary artery calcification in young adults: The Muscatine Study. *J Am Coll Cardiol* 1996;27:277-284.

6. Williams CL Hayman LL, Daniels SR, et al: Cardiovascular health in childhood: a statement for health professionals from the committee on atherosclerosis, hypertension, and obesity in the young (AHOY), Council on Cardiovascular Disease in the Young, American Heart Association. *Circulation* 2002;106:143-160.

7. Greenland P, Gidding SS, Tracey RP: Commentary: Lifelong prevention of atherosclerosis: the critical importance of major risk factor exposures. *Int J Epidemiol* 2002;31:1129-1134.

8. Enos WF, Holmes RH, Beyer J: Coronary disease among United States soldiers killed in action in Korea: preliminary report. *JAMA* 1953;152:1090-1093.

9. Davis PH, Dawson JD, Riley WA, Lauer RM: Carotid intimal–medial thickness is related to cardiovascular risk factors measured from childhood through middle age: the Muscatine Study. *Circulation* 2001;104:2815-2819.

10. Li S, Chen W, Srinivasan SR, et al: Childhood cardiovascular risk factors and carotid vascular changes in adulthood: the Bogalusa Heart Study. *JAMA* 2003;290:2271-2276.

11. Raitakari OT, Juonala M, Kahonen M, et al: Cardiovascular risk factors in childhood and carotid intima-media thickness in

adulthood: the Cardiovascular Risk in Young Finns Study. *JAMA* 2003;290:2277-2283.

12.   Lauer RM, Lee J, Clarke WR: Factors affecting the relationship between childhood and adult cholesterol levels: the Muscatine Study. *Pediatrics* 1988;82:309-318.

13.   Lauer RM, Clarke WR: Use of cholesterol measurements in childhood for the prediction of adult hypercholesterolemia: the Muscatine Study. *JAMA* 1990;264:3034-3038.

14.   Webber LS, Srinivasan SR, Wattigney WA, et al: Tracking of serum lipids and lipoproteins from childhood to adulthood: the Bogalusa Heart Study. *Am J Epidemiol* 1991;133:884-899.

15.   Ogden CL, Carroll MD, Flegal KM: High body mass index for age among US children and adolescents, 2003-2006. *JAMA* 2008;229:2401-2405.

16.   Eaton DK, Kann L, Kinchen S, et al: Youth Risk Behavior Surveillance: United States, 2005. *MMWR Surveill Summ* 2006;55:1-108.

17.   Rask-Nissila L, Jokinen E, Terho P, et al: Neurological development of 5-year old children receiving a low-saturated fat, low-cholesterol diet since infancy: a randomized controlled trial. *JAMA* 2000;284:993-1000.

18.   The DISC Collaborative Research Group: The efficacy and safety of lowering dietary intake of total fat, saturated fat, and cholesterol in children with elevated LDL-cholesterol: the Dietary Intervention Study in Children (DISC). *JAMA* 1995;273:1429-1435.

19.   National Cholesterol Education Program: Highlights of the Report of the Expert Panel on Blood Cholesterol Levels in Children and Adolescents. *Pediatrics* 1992;89:495-501.

20.   Wiegman A, Hutten BA, de Groot E, et al: Efficacy and safety of statin therapy in children with familial hypercholesterolemia: a randomized controlled trial. *JAMA* 2004;292:331-337.

21.   Clauss SB, Holmes BA, Hopkins P, et al: Efficacy and safety of lovastatin therapy in adolescent girls with heterozygous familial hypercholesterolemia. *Pediatrics* 2005;116:682-688.

22.   Avis HJ, Vissers MN, Stein EA, et al: A systematic review and meta-analysis of statin therapy in children with familial hypercholesterolemia. *Arterioscler Thromb Vasc Biol* 2007;27:1803-1810.

23.   McCrindle BW, Urbina EM, Dennison BA, et al: Drug therapy of high-risk lipid abnormalities in children and adolescents. *Circulation* 2007;115:1948-1967.

24. Daniels SR, Greer FR and the Committee on Nutrition: Lipid screening and cardiovascular health in childhood. *Pediatrics* 2008;122:198-208.

25. American Academy of Pediatrics, Committee on Nutrition: Cholesterol in childhood. *Pediatrics* 1998;101(1 pt 1);141-147.

26. Kavey RE, Daniels SR, Lauer RM, et al: American Heart Association guidelines for primary prevention of atherosclerotic cardiovascular disease beginning in childhood. *Circulation* 2003;107:1562-1566 (published simultaneously in *J Pediatr* 2003;142:368-372).

27. Kavey RE, Allada V, Daniels SR, et al: Cardiovascular risk reduction in high-risk pediatric populations: a scientific statement from the American Heart Association Expert Panel on Population and Prevention Science; Councils on Cardiovascular Disease in the Young, Epidemiology and Prevention, Nutrition, Physical Activity and Metabolism, High Blood Pressure Research, Cardiovascular Nursing, and the Kidney in Heart Disease; and the Interdisciplinary Working Group on Quality of Care and Outcomes Research-endorsed by the American Academy of Pediatrics. *Circulation* 2006;114:2710-2738.

28. US Department of Health & Human Services, US Department of Agriculture: *Dietary Guidelines for Americans*, 6th ed. Washington, DC, US Government Printing Office, 2005.

29. Lichenstein AH, Deckelbaum RJ: American Heart Association Science Advisory. Stanol/sterol ester-containing foods and blood cholesterol levels; a statement for healthcare professionals from the Nutrition Committee of the Council on Nutrition, Physical Activity, and Metabolism of the American Heart Association. *Circulation* 2001;103:1177-1179.

30. Tammi A, Ronnemaa T, Miettinen TA, et al: Effects of gender, apolipoprotein E phenotype and cholesterol-lowering by plant stanol esters in children: the STRIP study. Special Turku Coronary Risk Factor Intervention Project. *Acta Pediatr* 2002;91:1155-1162.

31. Hayman LL, Meininger JC, Daniels SR, et al: Primary prevention of cardiovascular disease in nursing practice: focus on children and youth. A scientific statement from the American Heart Association Committee on Atherosclerosis, Hypertension, and Obesity in Youth of the Council on Cardiovascular Disease in the Young, Council on Cardiovascular Nursing, Council on Epidemiology and Prevention and Council on Nutrition, Physical Activity and Metabolism. *Circulation* 2007;116:344-357.

32.   Barlow SE and the Expert Committee: Expert committee recommendations regarding the prevention, assessment, and treatment of child and adolescent overweight and obesity: summary report. *Pediatrics* 2007;120:S164-192.

33.   National High Blood Pressure Education Program NIH: The fourth report on the diagnosis, evaluation, and treatment of high blood pressure in children and adolescents. *Pediatrics* 2004;114:555-576.

34.   Hayman LL, Williams CL, Daniels, SR, et al: Cardiovascular health promotion in the schools: a statement for health and education professionals and child health advocates from the Committee on Atherosclerosis, Hypertension and Obesity in Youth (AHOY) of the Council on Cardiovascular Disease in the Young, American Heart Association. *Circulation* 2004;110:2266-2275.

35.   Gidding SS, Dennison BA, Birch LL, et al: Dietary recommendations for children and adolescents: a guide for practitioners. Consensus statement from the American Heart Association. *Circulation* 2005;112:2061-2075.

36.   Strong WB, Malina RM, Blimkic CJR, et al: Evidence-based physical activity for school-aged youth. *J Pediatr* 2005;146:732-737.

37.   US Department of Health & Human Services: 2008 Physical activity guidelines for Americans. Available at www.health.gov/pa-guidelines. Accessed July 10, 2009.

38. Trost SG, Loprinzi PD: Exercise-promoting healthy lifestyles in children and adolescents. *J Clin Lipid* 2008;2:162-168.

39.   Institute of Medicine, committee on prevention of obesity in children and youth: Food and nutrition board and board on health promotion and disease prevention. *Preventing Childhood Obesity: Health in the Balance*. Washington, DC, National Academies Press, 2005.

40.   Hayman LL: Behavioral medicine across the life course: challenges and opportunities for interdisciplinary science. *Ann Behavioral Med* 2007;33:236-241.

41.   Estabrooks PA, Fisher EB, Hayman LL: What is needed to reverse the trends in childhood obesity: a call to action. *Ann Behavioral Med* 2008;36:209-216.

42.   Fitzgibbon ML, Hayman LL, Haire-Joshu D: Childhood obesity: Can policy changes affect this epidemic? Society of Behavioral Medicine, 2008. Available at http://www.sbm.org/policy/childhoodobesity.asp. Accessed July 10, 2009.

Chapter 12

Acculturation and Coronary Heart Disease

By C. Tissa Kappagoda, MD, PhD,
and Ezra A. Amsterdam, MD

Acculturation is a process in which members of one cultural group adopt the beliefs and behaviors of another group. It "comprehends those phenomena which result when groups of individuals having different cultures come into continuous first-hand contact, with subsequent changes in the original culture patterns of either or both groups."[1] Although acculturation is usually in the direction of a minority group adopting habits and language patterns of the dominant group, it can be reciprocal—that is, the dominant group adopts patterns typical of the minority group. However, in the context of coronary heart disease (CHD), the effects are likely to be more evident in the minority group because assimilation often manifests by changes in dietary preferences (eg, a diet high in saturated fat), by adoption of new patterns of behavior (eg, lack of exercise and initiation of tobacco use), and by acceptance of body images (overweight) that are not necessarily consistent with promoting cardiovascular health. Apart from these factors, which predispose minorities to develop CHD, other issues that merit consideration are the beliefs pertaining to causation of disease and their impact on utilization of health-care services.

Measurement of Acculturation

Two instruments have been used in the United States to evaluate the extent of acculturation in Mexican-American populations: (a) Hazuda's scales developed for the San Antonio Heart Study[2] and (b) the Hispanic Health and Nutrition Examination Survey (HHANES), 1982-1984.[3] Both of these instruments (Table 12-1 and Table 12-2) show that their focus is only obliquely linked to matters pertaining to health care. They also illustrate one of the major issues in dealing with large minority groups whose only common feature is the language spoken in the new country. Both instruments focus on language as the main index of acculturation.[4] In practice, many studies have simply used the duration of time spent in the US as an index of acculturation. However, in contrast, a study of South Asian immigrants to the US who have lived here a median of 26 years, found that there was a disproportionately high prevalence of diabetes despite an above-average income and educational status. In this group, adherence to traditional beliefs was associated with diabetes with an odds ratio (OR) of 2.5 (Personal communication: Kanaya et al. Abstract presented at ADA Annual Session in San Francisco, 2008).

Acculturation and Mortality

One of the most compelling studies on this phenomenon was reported by Singh and Siapush.[5] They examined the extent to which various ethnic-immigrant and US-born groups differ in their risks of all-cause and cause-specific mortality, morbidity, and health behaviors. Using data from the National Longitudinal Mortality Study, 1979-1989, they estimated mortality risks of immigrants, relative to those of US-born individuals, for major US racial and ethnic groups. Compared with US-born whites of equivalent socioeconomic and demographic background, foreign-born blacks, Hispanics, and Asians/Pacific Islanders, US-born Asians/Pacific Islanders, US-born Hispanics,

Table 12-1: Items in the Final Acculturation and Structural Assimilation Scales

San Antonio Heart Study, San Antonio, Texas 1979-1982
Dimensions Measured, Scale Items, and Scale Score Ranges

Acculturation

I.   Early childhood experience with English versus Spanish language

    1. What was the first language you learned to speak?

    2. What language was spoken in your home when you were a child?

    Scale range: 2-6 points

II. Adult proficiency in English

    1. In your opinion, how well do you understand spoken English?

    2. In your opinion, how well do you speak English?

    3. In your opinion, how well do you read English?

    Scale range: 3-12 points

and foreign-born whites had, respectively, 48%, 45%, 43%, 32%, 26%, and 16% lower (all-cause) mortality risks. While American Indians did not differ significantly from US-born whites, US-born blacks had an 8% higher mortality risk. Black and Hispanic immigrants experi-

III. Adult pattern of English versus Spanish language usage

1. What language do you usually use with your spouse?

2. What language do you usually use with your children?

3. What language do you usually use with your parents?

4. What language do you usually use at family gatherings, such as Christmas or other holidays?

5. What language do you usually use with most of your friends?

6. What language do you usually with most of your neighbors?

7. What language do you usually use with most of the people at work?

8. In what language are the TV programs you watch?

9. In what language are the radio stations you listen to?

10. In what language are the books and magazines you read?

Scale range: 10-50 points

(continued on next page) 12

enced, respectively, 52% and 26%, lower mortality risks than their US-born counterparts (Table 12-3).

Considerable differentials were also found in mortality for cardiovascular disease with Asian/Pacific Islanders and Hispanic immigrants generally experiencing the low-

Table 12-1: Items in the Final Acculturation and Structural Assimilation Scales *(continued)*

San Antonio Heart Study, San Antonio, Texas 1979-1982
Dimensions Measured, Scale Items, and Scale Score Ranges

Acculturation (continued)

IV. Value placed on preserving Mexican cultural origin

1. How important do you feel it is for your children to know something about the history of Mexico?

2. How important do you feel it is for your children to follow Mexican customs and ways of life?

3. How important do you feel it is for your children to celebrate Mexican holidays such as Cinco de Mayo or El Diez y Seis de Septiembre?

Scale range: 3-15 points

V. Attitude toward traditional family structure and sex-role organization

1. Knowing your family ancestry or lineage, that is, tracing your family tree, is an important part of family life.

2. It is important to know your cousins, aunts, and uncles and to have a close relationship with them.

3. A person should remember other family members who have passed away on the anniversary of their death, All Soul's Day, or other special occasions.

4. Brothers have a responsibility to protect their sisters while they are growing up.

5. While they are growing up, sisters have an obligation to respect their brother's authority.

6. If they could live anywhere they wanted to, married children should live close to their parents so that they can help each other.

7. In the absence of the father, the most important decisions should be made by the eldest son rather than the mother, if the son is old enough.

Scale range: 7-35 points

Structural Assimilation

I. Childhood interaction with members of mainstream society

1. When you were growing up, were your neighbors mostly Mexican American, mostly Anglo, or about equal numbers of each?

2. When you were growing up, were your schoolmates mostly Mexican American, mostly Anglo, or about equal numbers of each?

3. When you were growing up, were your close, personal friends mostly Mexican American, mostly Anglo, or about equal numbers of each?

Scale range: 3-9 points

12

(continued on next page)

Table 12-1: Items in the Final Acculturation and Structural Assimilation Scales *(continued)*

San Antonio Heart Study, San Antonio, Texas 1979-1982
Dimensions Measured, Scale Items, and Scale Score Ranges

Structural Assimilation (continued)

II. Adult interaction with members of mainstream society

1. Throughout your adult life, have your neighbors been mostly Mexican American, mostly Anglo, or about equal numbers of each?

2. Throughout your adult life, have your close, personal friends been mostly Mexican American, mostly Anglo, or about equal numbers of each?

3. Are the people with whom you work closely on the job/Are the people with whom you worked closely on your last job mostly Mexican American, mostly Anglo, or about equal numbers of each?

Scale range: 3-9 points

---

est risks. Consistent with the acculturation hypothesis, immigrants' risks of smoking, obesity, hypertension, and other chronic conditions, although substantially lower than those for the US born, increased with increasing length of US residence (Table 12-4).

This study showed considerable variations in mortality patterns for immigrants and those born in the US, with immigrants in each major racial/ethnic group showing a significantly lower risk of mortality than their native-born counterparts, even after controlling for a number of socioeconomic and demographic factors. Mortality differentials between immigrants and the US born are larg-

Table 12-2: Hispanic Health and Nutrition Examination Survey (HHANES), 1982-1984

1. What language do you speak?

2. What language do you prefer?

3. What language do you read better?

4. What language do you write better?

5. What ethnic identification do you use?

6. What ethnic identification does/did your mother use?

7. What ethnic identification does/did you father use?

8. Where was the birthplace of yourself, your mother, your father?

est for blacks and Hispanics. Although blacks have been generally shown to have twice the mortality level (before adjusting for socioeconomic differences) of whites, a very different pattern emerges when they are stratified by nativity status. Black immigrants have the lowest mortality of all ethnic-nativity groups and their mortality risk is half of that of US-born whites. US-born black women but not men retain a significantly higher mortality risk than their comparable US-born white counterparts. The same applies to Asians/Pacific Islanders and Hispanics.

The mortality advantage of ethnic immigrants appears to be even greater among those of working age. Ethnic-nativity differentials in mortality for cardiovascular disease were generally similar to those for the overall mortality, and Hispanic, Asians/Pacific Islanders, and black immigrants exhibited the lowest cardiovascular disease risks (Table 12-3).

Table 12-3: Adjusted Mortality Differentials in Ethnic Immigrants >18 Years

Covariate	Both Sexes	
	RR	95% CI
	Aged 25-64 Years	
Ethnic-Nativity Group		
US-born, non-Hispanic white	1.00	**Reference**
Foreign-born, non-Hispanic white	0.74[b]	0.67, 0.83
US-born, black	1.25[b]	1.18, 1.32
Foreign-born, black	0.52[b]	0.31, 0.86
US-born, Asian and Pacific Islander	0.77[a]	0.62, 0.97
Foreign-born, Asian and Pacific Islander	0.55[b]	0.43, 0.71
US-born, Hispanic	0.73[b]	0.64, 0.84
Foreign-born, Hispanic	0.48[b]	0.41, 0.57
American Indian	1.28[b]	1.07, 1.54
Sample size	244,925	

[a]$P <0.05$, [b]$P <0.01$. RR=relative risk (hazard ratio), CI=confidence interval

Data taken from Singh et al[5]

Reference=indicates subgroup against which others were compared

Hispanics

Data from the NHANES survey (1988-1994) have provided some interesting information about the effect of one probable index of acculturation among Mexican

Men		Women	
RR	95% CI	RR	95% CI
Aged 25-64 Years			
1.00	**Reference**	1.00	**Reference**
0.72[b]	0.63, 0.83	0.76[b]	0.65, 0.90
1.25[b]	1.16, 1.34	1.26[b]	1.15, 1.37
0.66	0.37, 1.20	0.32[b]	0.12, 0.86
0.75[a]	0.56, 0.99	0.81	0.56, 1.16
0.51[b]	0.36, 0.71	0.61[b]	0.43, 0.88
0.75[b]	0.63, 0.89	0.71[b]	0.57, 0.89
0.55[b]	0.45, 0.68	0.38[b]	0.28, 0.52
1.16	0.91, 1.48	1.48[b]	1.11, 1.96
117,796		127,129	

Reference=indicates subgroup against which others were compared

(continued on next page)

Americans living in the US, which was the language spoken.[6] Data from this national sample (1988-1994)—of 1,387 Mexican-American women and 1,404 Mexican-American men (25 to 64 years)—were examined to

Table 12-3: Adjusted Mortality Differentials in Ethnic Immigrants >18 Years *(Continued)*

Covariate	Both Sexes	
	RR	95% CI
	Aged 65+ Years	
Ethnic-Nativity Group		
US-born, non-Hispanic white	1.00	**Reference**
Foreign-born, non-Hispanic white	0.87[b]	0.83, 0.92
US-born, black	0.92[b]	0.88, 0.97
Foreign-born, black	0.55[b]	0.37, 0.82
US-born, Asian and Pacific Islander	0.55[b]	0.41, 0.73
Foreign-born, Asian and Pacific Islander	0.57[b]	0.47, 0.69
US-born, Hispanic	0.73[b]	0.63, 0.85
Foreign-born, Hispanic	0.59[b]	0.51, 0.68
American Indian	0.87	0.70, 1.08
Sample size	55,985	

[a]$P < 0.05$, [b]$P < 0.01$. RR=relative risk (hazard ratio), CI=confidence interval

Data taken from Singh et al[5]

Reference=indicates subgroup against which others were compared

estimate CHD mortality risk and five primary cardiovascular disease risk factors: systolic blood pressure, body mass index (BMI), cigarette smoking, non-high-density lipoprotein cholesterol, and type 2 diabetes. Differences

	Men		Women	
	RR	95% CI	RR	95% CI
		Aged 65+ Years		
	1.00	**Reference**	1.00	**Reference**
	0.84[b]	0.78, 0.90	0.91[b]	0.85, 0.97
	0.85[b]	0.79, 0.92	0.99	0.92, 1.07
	0.41[b]	0.22, 0.76	0.74	0.45, 1.23
	0.55[b]	0.38, 0.79	0.55[b]	0.35, 0.87
	0.57[b]	0.45, 0.72	0.56[b]	0.41, 0.77
	0.67[b]	0.55, 0.81	0.83	0.66, 1.04
	0.54[b]	0.44, 0.66	0.65[b]	0.53, 0.80
	0.80	0.59, 1.09	0.91	0.68, 1.23
	23,355		32,630	

12

Reference=indicates subgroup against which others were compared

in risk were evaluated by country of birth and primary language spoken.

The estimated 10-year CHD mortality risk per 1,000 persons, adjusted for age and education, was highest for

Table 12-4: Risk Factors and Acculturation as Measured by Time in the US[5]

Covariate	Cigarette Smoking		Obesity		Hypertension		Chronic Condition	
	OR	95% CI	OR	95% CI	OR	95% CI	OR	95% CI
Ethnic-Nativity Group								
US-born, non-Hispanic white	1.00	Reference	1.00	Reference	1.00	Reference	1.00	Reference
Foreign-born, non-Hispanic white	0.96	0.84, 1.10	0.85[b]	0.79, 0.91	0.84[a]	0.73, 0.97	0.73[b]	0.69, 0.77
US-born, black	0.78[b]	0.72, 0.84	1.87[b]	1.80, 1.94	1.82[b]	1.67, 1.98	0.84[b]	0.81, 0.87
Foreign-born, black	0.25[b]	0.17, 0.36	1.07	0.93, 1.22	1.38[a]	1.02, 1.85	0.52[b]	0.45, 0.59
US-born, Asian and Pacific Islander	0.89	0.65, 1.21	0.66[b]	0.56, 0.78	1.53[b]	1.12, 2.10	0.73[b]	0.64, 0.83
Foreign-born, Asian and Pacific Islander	0.54[b]	0.45, 0.65	0.28[b]	0.25, 0.32	0.62[b]	0.50, 0.77	0.44[b]	0.41, 0.48

	OR	CI	OR	CI	OR	CI	OR	CI
US-born, Hispanic	0.59[b]	0.52, 0.67	1.44[b]	1.36, 1.53	1.10	0.95, 1.28	0.80[b]	0.76, 0.85
Foreign-born, Hispanic	0.37[b]	0.32, 0.43	1.11[b]	1.05, 1.18	0.78[b]	0.67, 0.91	0.47[b]	0.45, 0.50
American Indian	1.40[b]	1.10, 1.77	1.66[b]	1.47, 1.87	1.86[b]	1.43, 2.43	1.04	0.92, 1.17
Duration of Residence Since the Time of Immigration to the US								
<1 yr	0.48[b]	0.30, 0.79	0.39[b]	0.29, 0.52	0.34[b]	0.15, 0.75	0.44[b]	0.36, 0.55
1-5 yr	0.67[b]	0.53, 0.84	0.62[b]	0.55, 0.69	0.67[b]	0.50, 0.91	0.48[b]	0.44, 0.53
5-10 yr	0.68[b]	0.55, 0.83	0.65[b]	0.59, 0.72	0.65[b]	0.50, 0.85	0.52[b]	0.47, 0.57
10-15 yr	0.64[b]	0.52, 0.80	0.72[b]	0.65, 0.79	0.75[a]	0.59, 0.97	0.61[b]	0.56, 0.67
15+ year	0.82[b]	0.72, 0.92	0.87[b]	0.83, 0.92	0.81[b]	0.71, 0.91	0.76[b]	0.72, 0.79
US born	1.00	Reference	1.00	Reference	1.00	Reference	1.00	Reference
Sample size	40,373		161,134		40,279		162,516	

Table is adjusted for age, sex, race/ethnicity, nativity, marital status, family size, place, and region of residence, education, employment status, and family income. [a]P <0.05, [b]P <0.01. CI=confidence interval, OR=odds ratio

Source: Derived from the National Health Interview Survey, 1993-1994

Reference=indicates subgroup against which others were compared

12

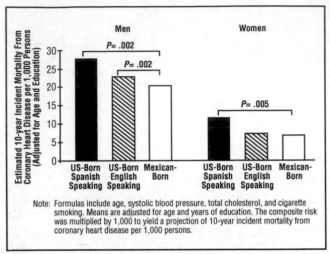

Figure 12-1: Estimated 10-year risk of mortality from coronary artery disease, according to gender-specific formulas based on the National Health and Nutrition Survey (1988-1994) data.[6]

US-born Spanish-speaking men and women (27.5 and 11.4, respectively), intermediate for US-born English-speaking men and women (22.5 and 7.0), and lowest for Mexican-born men and women (20.0 and 6.6) (Figure 12-1). A similar pattern of higher risk among US-born Spanish-speaking men and women was demonstrated for each of the 5 cardiovascular disease risk factors (Table 12-5). The authors concluded that "the distinct cardiovascular risk profile of US-born Spanish-speaking Mexican Americans may have lost some of the advantages associated with the Mexican lifestyle without gaining the advantages associated with acculturation into the English-speaking culture," at least with respect to CHD. This conclusion was supported by the findings in Hispanics in the Multi-Ethnic Study of Atherosclerosis (MESA) study, where after adjustment for age and gender, Spanish-speaking

Hispanics with cardiovascular risk factors had higher systolic blood pressure, fasting low-density lipoprotein (LDL) cholesterol, and fasting blood glucose compared to English-speaking Hispanics.[7]

The MESA study also provided insights into the effect of acculturation on subclinical CHD as measured by coronary calcification.[8] As mentioned previously, the study cohort consisted of 2,553 non-Hispanic whites, 1,734 non-Hispanic blacks, 1,457 Hispanics, and 797 Chinese residing in the US. Coronary calcium was assessed by chest CT. Being foreign born was associated with a lower prevalence of coronary calcification in blacks (relative prevalence [RP], 0.75) and in Hispanics (RP, 0.89) after adjustment for age, sex, income, and education. Years in the US were positively associated with prevalence of calcification in non–US-born Chinese (adjusted RP per 10 years in US, 1.06) and non–US-born blacks (RP, 1.59). Low educational level was associated with a higher prevalence of calcification in whites but with lower prevalence in Hispanics (RP, 0.91). US birth and time in the US were also positively associated with the extent of calcification in persons with detectable coronary calcium. These differences did not appear to be accounted for by smoking, BMI, LDL cholesterol, high-density lipoprotein (HDL) cholesterol, hypertension, and diabetes. The authors concluded that acculturation, as defined by years in the US and socioeconomic factors, is associated with differences in the prevalence and amount of coronary calcification in whites, Chinese, blacks, and Hispanics. Substantially similar conclusions were arrived at in a parallel study on the MESA cohort where carotid plaque was examined as a marker for subclinical atherosclerosis.[9]

Asians

Diet is perhaps the factor most significantly influenced by acculturation in minority populations. A recent study examined the dietary habits of 244 women of Chinese

Table 12-5: Cardiovascular Risk Factors by Migration and Acculturation Status and Education Level for Hispanic Women and Men Aged 25-64 Years (NHANES III 1988-1994)[6]

Group	SBP (mm Hg)	Mean BMI (kg/m²)
Women		
Mexican born	113.6	27.8
US born, English speaking	114.5	29.1
US born, Spanish speaking	119.5	29.7
White, non-Hispanic	113.0	26.3
Men		
Mexican born	118.6	26.9
US born, English speaking	121.5	28.1
US born, Spanish speaking	123.9	28.0
White, non-Hispanic	120.5	27.0

BMI=body mass index, SBP=systolic blood pressure

ethnicity living in Seattle, WA, and Vancouver, Canada.[10] Participants generally believed that there were strong relationships between diet and health, but only about a quarter were aware of nutrition information from the corresponding government. The respondents' older relatives and spouses who tended to prefer a Chinese diet had a

Current Smoker (%)	Non-HDL Chol (mg/dL)	Diabetes Mellitus (%)
11.6	146.6	6.9
18.2	148.6	6.1
20.4	154.7	13.5
30.1	149.0	4.2
32.8	159.8	5.0
27.5	159.8	7.1
33.6	158.8	13.4
33.3	161.0	4.8

Means and % values are adjusted for age and education.
Non-HDL Chol=non-high-density lipoprotein cholesterol

12

strong influence on the household diet and those with such family pressures ate more fruits and vegetables (4.4 vs 3.7 servings daily). In this context, older, less educated respondents considered it very important to eat a low fat, high fruit and vegetable diet. Younger, more educated participants who were employed outside the home did not think the (traditional) Chinese diet was healthier than a typical Western diet (all P <0.05). Such Western acculturated respondents were cognizant of nutrition information from the government and were more likely to believe in a relationship between diet and cancer/heart disease, and those with this knowledge increased fruit and vegetable consumption after immigration (all P <0.05). The authors made the point that traditional health beliefs, as well as socioeconomic and environmental factors related to diet, should be incorporated into the design and implementation of culturally appropriate health promotion programs for Chinese immigrants.

The diet of Japanese Americans has been investigated in greater depth than that of any other immigrant group in the US. Several descriptive studies have addressed this issue. Nisei (second-generation Japanese Americans, the offspring of immigrants) consumed greater amounts of tofu, rice, soy sauce, fish, tsukemono (pickled vegetables), and butter or margarine than did Sansei (third-generation Japanese Americans, the offspring of Nisei). The Sansei subjects, who presumably were more acculturated to a Western lifestyle, were more frequent consumers of cheese, salty snacks, and soft drinks than were the Nisei.[11,12] In contrast, a third study showed that Japanese persons living in Japan consume more fish, eggs, and soy products (tofu included) and less animal meats and dairy than do Japanese Americans.[13] These descriptive studies suggested that consumption of specific foods signified dietary acculturation in Japanese Americans. Against this background, Pierce al[14] used confirmatory factor analysis (CFA) to detect dietary patterns associated with traditional Japanese and Western diets in a community-based sample of Nisei and Sansei persons and their link with diabetes status and two risk factors for diabetes—BMI and C-reactive protein (CRP).

This study, which was done on a cross-sectional sample of 219 Nisei (mean age 70 years) and 277 Sansei (mean age 42 years), focused on CFA on five items characteristic of a Japanese diet and four items characteristic of a Western diet. The Nisei had a significantly higher average score for the Japanese food factor and significantly lower average score for the Western food factor than did the Sansei. In Sansei persons, but not in Nisei, the Western food factor score was significantly associated with plasma CRP concentration ($P=0.02$), BMI ($P=0.02$), and diabetes ($P=0.001$). It was suggested that the level of acculturation could influence at least one putative cardiovascular risk factor.[14]

Besides diet, the effect of acculturation on the prevalence of cardiovascular disease in Japanese Americans has also been extensively investigated. Some of the early data showed an east to west gradient in prevalence from Japan through Hawaii to California.[15] However, the Honolulu Heart Study re-examined this idea, having excluded subjects with prevalent disease and focused instead on the incidence. In a cohort of 4,653 men of Japanese ancestry living in Hawaii, with traditional Japanese social and cultural lifestyles, two of four scales of acculturation were significantly associated with CHD prevalence independently of 11 other risk factors, but none of the acculturation scales was associated with incidence. This apparent discrepancy is perhaps due to problems designating differences between angina and true myocardial infarction (MI). Measures of acculturation were also significantly associated with many of the other CHD risk factors in such a way that the more traditional Japanese men had lower serum cholesterol and uric acid levels, were less obese, more physically active, and smoked fewer cigarettes than the more Westernized men.[16]

The California Health Interview Survey in 2001 examined the effects of ethnicity, nativity (Spanish, Chinese, Vietnamese, Korean, and Khmer and Asian Indians), and years in the US on leisure time physical activity, nonleisure time physical activity, and occupational physical activity.[17] A total of 4,226 Asian Americans and 29,473 US-born non-Asians were included. Both male and female Asian Americans were much less likely to meet recommended levels of leisure time physical activity than US-born non-Asians (OR men=0.51, OR women=0.48). Foreign-born Asians were least likely to participate in leisure time physical activity, which increased with time spent in the US. After accounting for nonleisure time physical activity, Asian Americans had significantly lower estimated weekly energy expenditures than US-born non-Asians. These findings were corroborated in a study in Chinese-American children (8-10 years of age) whose cardiovascular risk factors were worse depending on the paternal level of acculturation.[18] A low level of physical activity and high paternal BMI were associated with higher systolic blood pressure and higher LDL levels in children.

Cigarette smoking is the most preventable risk factor for many negative health consequences, including cancer, heart disease, and lung disease. In the US, the prevalence rate of smoking is approximately 22%. This rate tends to be higher (26%-70%) in Asian immigrants, with Southeast Asian men having the highest rate. The effect of acculturation on smoking has been estimated in several studies in this group. A meta-analysis based on nine studies (1994 through 2005) has shown that, overall, there was no significant difference in the prevalence of cigarette smoking between acculturated and traditional Asian Americans (men, women, and adolescents).[4] However, acculturated men were 53% less likely to smoke than non-acculturated or "traditional" men, while acculturated women were 5 times more likely to smoke than traditional women. Adolescent Asians on average were almost 2 times more likely to smoke than traditional adolescents. Thus, it appeared that acculturation had a protective effect on smoking behavior in Asian men and a harmful effect in Asian women and adolescents. The overall magnitude of the effect was larger in women and adolescents than in men. However, these findings have to be viewed against a background of a higher prevalence of smoking in men compared to women.[19]

Also of interest, the prevalence of self-reported psychosocial stress is less in Asian immigrants to the US compared to their white counterparts. However, this "advantage" appeared to be attenuated in proportion to the time spent in the US.[20]

As Choi et al[4] observed, acculturation to US society may represent breaking away from traditional norms in Asian culture and adopting behaviors that are considered appropriate in the US culture. Although traditional social norms in Asian culture discourage women from smoking, US culture promotes more independence and equality in women's roles, including permissibility of women's smoking, possibly leading to increased smoking among acculturated women. Conversely, Asian men may be subjected to greater social pressures at work and in public places to quit smoking than would be true of men in Asian countries, which contributes to decreased smoking among acculturated men.

In the context of lifestyle-related changes, the Konkani Heart Study,[21] which focused on a community of immigrants from the west coast of India, established that alcohol consumption was a cardiac risk factor in this group. This factor acquired importance as the time spent in the US increased. The authors suggested that alcohol may have altered insulin resistance in a manner that promoted the occurrence of the metabolic syndrome and diabetes.

Summary

An issue that merits comment is the potentially confounding effects of acculturation and ethnicity. The issue is particularly important in evaluating differences between Hispanic populations and other ethnic groups, especially when the relative proportions of US-born and foreign-born Hispanics are not stipulated. The application of the Framingham model for prediction of risk for CHD is possibly an example of the validity of this suggestion. Application of the general gender-specific Framingham model to the constituents of a mixed American population systematically overestimated the 5-year incidence of coronary death and MI in Japanese, Hispanic American men, and native American women while it predicted those in white Americans and African Americans. However, after recalibration, the original equations predicted events accurately.[22]

References

1.   Redfield R, Linton R, Herskovits MJ: Memorandum for the study of acculturation. *Am Anthropol* 1936;38:149-152.

2.   Hazuda HP, Stern MP, Haffner SM: Acculturation and assimilation among Mexican Americans: scales and population-based data. *Soc Sc Q* 1988;69:687-706.

3.   Solis JM, Marks G, Garcia M, Shelton D: Acculturation, access to care, and use of preventive services by Hispanics: findings from HHANES 1982-84. *Am J Public Health* 1990;80:(suppl):11-19.

4.   Choi S, Rankin S, Stewart A, Oka R: Effects of acculturation on smoking behavior in Asian Americans: a meta-analysis. *J Cardiovasc Nurs* 2008;23:67-73.

5.   Singh GK, Siahpush M: Ethnic-immigrant differentials in health behaviors, morbidity, and cause-specific mortality in the United States: an analysis of two national data bases. *Hum Biol* 2002;74:83-109.

6.   Sundquist J, Winkleby MA: Cardiovascular risk factors in Mexican American adults: a transcultural analysis of NHANES III, 1988-1994. *Am J Public Health* 1999;89:723-730.

7.   Eamranond PP, Legedza AT, Diez Roux AV, et al: Association between language and risk factor levels among Hispanic adults with hypertension, hypercholesterolemia, or diabetes. *Am Heart J* 2009;157:53-59.

8.   Diez Roux AV, Detrano R, Jackson S, et al: Acculturation and socioeconomic position as predictors of coronary calcification in a multiethnic sample. *Circulation* 2005;112:1557-1565.

9.   Lutsey PL, Diez Roux AV, Jacobs DR Jr, et al: Associations of acculturation and socioeconomic status with subclinical cardiovascular disease in the multi-ethnic study of atherosclerosis. *Am J Public Health* 2008;98:1963-1970.

10.   Satia-Abouta J, Patterson RE, Kristal AR, et al: Psychosocial predictors of diet and acculturation in Chinese American and Chinese Canadian women. *Ethn Health* 2002;7:21-39.

11.   Kudo Y, Falciglia G, Couch SC: Evolution of meal patterns and food choices of Japanese-American females born in the United States. *Eur J Clin Nutr* 2000;54:665-670.

12.   Nakamura M, Whitlock G, Aoki N, et al: Japanese and Western diet and risk of idiopathic sudden deafness: a case-control study using pooled controls. *Int J Epidemiol* 2001;30:608-615.

13.   Takata Y, Maskarinec G, Franke A, et al: A comparison of dietary habits among women in Japan and Hawaii. *Public Health Nutr* 2004;7:319-326.

14.   Pierce BL Austin MA, Crane PK, et al: Measuring dietary acculturation in Japanese Americans with the use of confirmatory factor analysis of food-frequency data. *Am J Clin Nutr* 2007;86:496-503.

15.   Marmot MG, Syme SL, Kagan A, et al: Epidemiologic studies of coronary heart disease and stroke in Japanese men living in Japan, Hawaii and California: prevalence of coronary and hypertensive disease and associated risk factors. *Am J Epidemiol* 1975;102:514-525.

16.   Reed D, McGee D, Cohen J, et al: Acculturation and coronary heart disease among Japanese men in Hawaii. *Am J Epidemiol* 1982;115:894-905.

17.   Kandula N, Lauderdale DS: Leisure time, non-leisure time, and occupational physical activity in Asian Americans. *Ann Epidemiol* 2005;15:257-265.

18.   Chen JL, Wu Y: Cardiovascular risk factors in Chinese American children: associations between overweight, acculturation, and physical activity. *J Pediatr Health Care* 2008;22:103-110.

19.   Tsai YW, Tsai TI, Yang CL, Kuo KN: Gender differences in smoking behaviors in an Asian population. *J Womens Health (Larchmt)* 2008;17:971-978.

20.   Uppaluri CR, Schumm LP, Lauderdale DS: Self-reports of stress in Asian immigrants: effects of ethnicity and acculturation. *Ethn Dis* 2001;11:107-14.

12

21.   Mooteri SN, Petersen F, Dagubati R, Pai RG: Duration of residence in the United States as a new risk factor for coronary artery disease (The Konkani Heart Study). *Am J Cardiol* 2004;93:359-361.

22.   D'Agostino RB Sr, Grundy S, et al, and the CHD Risk Prediction Group: Validation of the Framingham coronary heart disease prediction scores: results of a multiple ethnic groups investigation. *JAMA* 2001;286:180-187.

Appendix A

Summary of 2008 Update on Heart Disease and Stroke Statistics: A Report From the American Heart Association Statistics Committee and Stroke Statistics Committee[1]

Figures were calculated from mortality rates for 2004 and for disease and risk factor prevalence; most rates were calculated from the 1999-2004 National Health and Nutrition Examination Survey (NHANES).

Sources and dates are included with all headings.

Abbreviations: AmInd=American Indian and Alaskan; MexAm=Mexican American; F=female; M=male; ARIC=Atherosclerosis Risk in Communities Study; BRFSS=Behavioral Risk Factor Surveillance System; CDC=Centers for Disease Control and Prevention; CHS= Cardiovascular Health Study; FHS=Framingham Heart Study; MEPS=Medical Expenditure Panel Survey; NCHS=National Center for Health Statistics; NHIS=National Health Interview Survey; NHLBI=National Heart, Lung and Blood Institute; YRBS= Youth Risk Behavior Surveillance

1. Cardiovascular Disease

A. *Cardiovascular disease (CVD) prevalence % (≥18 years) (NHIS, NCHS 2005, NHANES, NHLBI)*

	CVD	HD	CHD	Stroke	Hypertension
White	12.0	6.6	2.3	21.0	
M	37.2				
F	35.0				
Black		10.2	6.2	3.4	31.2
M	44.6				
F	49.0				
Hispanic MexAm		8.3	5.9	2.2	20.3
M	31.6				
F	34.4				
Asian		6.7	3.8	2.0	19.4
AmInd		13.0	2.5	5.8	25.5

HD=heart disease; CHD=coronary heart disease

B. *2004 overall death rates for CVD (per 100,000)*

White		Black	
M	335.1	M	454.0
F	238.0	F	333.6

AmInd*		Hispanic*	
M	182.7	M	193.9
F	119.9	F	130.0

*HD only

C. 2004 age-adjusted mortality rates for CHD and stroke: Females (NCHS, NHLBI)

	CHD	Stroke
White	114.7	47.2
Black	148.7	65.5

D. 2004 selected causes of death, % (NCHS, NHLBI)

		CVD	Cancer	Diabetes
White	M	35.1	24.6	2.8
	F	37.7	22.0	-
Black	M	32.9	22.2	3.8
	F	38.1	21.3	5.1
Hispanic	M	26.5	19.0	4.1
	F	30.4	21.4	
Asian	M	32.9	26.7	3.3
	F	33.5	26.9	-
AmInd	M	23.6	17.4	4.5
	F	25.0	19.2	4.2

(continued on next page)

1. Cardiovascular Disease *(continued)*

E. *Highest prevalences of risk factors (BRFSS, CDC)*

Obesity: Hispanic males with
high school education   29.7%

Black women ±
high school education   48.4%

Hypertension:
Blacks   41.2%

F. *Healthy lifestyle (MEPS, 2004)*

Moderate to vigorous physical activity:

Non-Hispanic white	58.5%
Non-Hispanic black	52.5%
Hispanic	51.4%
All men	60.3%
All women	53.1%

Nonsmokers:

Hispanics	84.2%
Non-Hispanic white	77.8%
Non-Hispanic black	76.3%
All men	75.7%
All women	81.7%

2. Coronary Heart Disease

A. Incidence (ARIC): 45-64 years; age-adjusted/1,000 person-years

White	M	12.5	Black	M	10.6
	F	4.0		F	5.1

First MI (1987-2001): rate/1,000

White	M	3.9	Black	M	4.2
	F	1.7		F	2.8

B. Prevalence % (≥20 years) 2005 (NHANES, NCHS, NHLBI, NHIS)

		CHD	MI
Non-Hispanic WM		9.4	5.4
Non-Hispanic WF		6.0	2.5
Black M		7.1	3.9
Black F		7.8	3.3
MexAm M		5.6	3.1
MexAm F		5.3	2.1
Hispanic (M&F)	≥18	5.9	
Asian	≥18	3.8	
AmInd	≥18	2.5	

MI=myocardial infarction

(continued on next page)

2. Coronary Heart Disease *(continued)*

C. Risk factor predictors for CHD

		Hypertension	Diabetes
White	M	1.6	2.0
	F	2.1	3.3
Black	M	2.0	1.6
	F	4.8	1.8

D. CHD mortality (per 100,000) (FHS, NHLBI)

White	M	192.4	Hispanic	119.2
	F	114.7	Asian	84.1
Black	M	223.9	AmInd	06.5
	F	148.7		

E. Post-MI mortality % (FHS, ARIC, CHS)

		Within 1 Year	Within 5 years
40-69 years			
White	M	8	15
	F	12	22
Black	M	14	27
	F	11	32
≥70 years			
White	M	27	50
	F	32	56
Black	M	26	56
	F	28	62

3. Stroke

A. Incidence (45-84 years; age-adjusted/1,000 population)

White	M	3.6	Black	M	6.6
	F	2.3		F	4.9

First ever stroke (1993-1994, 1999)[2] (per 100,000)		Ischemic	Intercerebral Hemorrhage	Subarachnoid Hemorrhage
White	1993-94	156	20	6
	1999	181	24	7
Black	1993-94	226	42	11
	1999	219	44	11

B. Prevalence % (≥20 years) (NHIS, 2005)

White	M	2.4
	F	2.7
Black	M	4.1
	F	4.1
AmInd	≥18 years	5.8
Asian	≥18 years	2.0
Hispanic	≥18 years	2.2

C. 2005 stroke mortality (per 100,000) (NCHS)

White M	48.1	White F	47.2
Black M	74.9	Black F	65.5
Hispanic M	41.5	Hispanic F	35.4
Asian M	44.2	Asian F	38.9
AmInd M	35.0	AmInd F	35.1

4. Hypertension

A. Prevalence %, ≥20 years (NHANES 1999-2004, NCHS, NHLBI)

White	M	32.5
	F	31.9
Black	M	42.6
	F	46.6
MexAm	M	28.7
	F	31.4
Hispanic	≥18 years	20.3
Asian	≥18 years	19.4
AmInd	≥18 years	25.5

B. Prevalence increase (1988-1994 to 1999-2002)[3]

White	24.3% to 28.1%
Black	35.8% to 41.4%

C. Hypertension related mortality: Age-standardized per 100,000 population (1995-2002 CDC)

Non-Hispanic White		135.9
Hispanic	M	135.9
	F	118.3

D. 2004 hypertension mortality rate (NCHS, NHLBI)

White	M	15.7
	F	14.5
Black	M	51.0
	F	40.9

5. Congenital Heart Disease

A. Prevalence, % of total (2002)[4] (excludes bicuspid aortic valve)

	Children	Adults
Ventricular septal defect	20.1	20.1
Atrial septal defect	16.8	20.6
Patent ductus arteriosus	12.4	16.3
Valvular pulmonic stenosis	12.6	14.4
Coarctation of aorta	6.8	8.4
Tetralogy of Fallot	7.0	5.4
Valvular aortic stenosis	5.5	5.2
Total	81.2	90.4

B. Mortality: crude infant death rates (per 100,000) (CDC, 2004)

White infants	38.3
Black infants	56.0

6. Heart Failure

A. Prevalence %, age ≥20 years (NHANES 1999-2004, NHLBI)

White	M	2.8
	F	2.1
Black	M	2.7
	F	3.3
MexAm	M	2.1
	F	1.9

7. Smoking/Tobacco Use

A. Use of any tobacco product % (NCHS, 2004)

White	31.4
Black	27.3
Hispanic	23.3
Asian	11.7
AmInd	33.8

B. Cigarette smokers % (2005) (≥18 years) (NHIS, NCHS)

White	M	24.0
	F	20.0
Black	M	26.7
	F	17.3
Hispanic	M	21.1
	F	11.1
Asian	M	20.6
	F	6.1
AmInd	M	37.5
	F	26.8

C. Youth cigarette smokers %, grades 9-12 (YRBS, CDC, 2005)

White	M	24.9
	F	27.0
Black	M	14.0
	F	11.9
Hispanic	M	24.8
	F	19.2

8. Blood Cholesterol

A. Total cholesterol levels, 12-19 years (NHANES 2003-2004, NCHS)

		mg/dL
White	M	157.1
	F	167.5
Black	M	161.3
	F	162.7
MexAm	M	159.6
	F	161.4

B. LDL cholesterol levels (NHANES 2003-2004, NCHS)

		12-19 years mg/dL	≥20years mg/dL
White	M	90.3	126
	F	91.5	121
Black	M	87.9	121
	F	91.4	121
MexAm	M	89.9	125
	F	92.0	117

(continued on next page)

8. Blood Cholesterol *(continued)*

C. HDL cholesterol levels (NHANES 2003-2004, NCHS)

		12-19 years mg/dL	≥20 years mg/dL
White	M	47.0	45.5
	F	56.5	56.6
Black	M	54.4	51.0
	F	57.6	57.3
MexAm	M	49.4	45.0
	F	53.7	52.9

D. 2005 Prevalence of categories of cholesterol, age ≥20 years, mg/dL by % of population (NHANES 1999-2004, BRFSS)

		Total cholesterol ≥200	≥240	LDL ≥130	HDL ≤40
White	M	47.9	16.1	31.7	26.2
	F	49.7	18.2	33.8	8.8
Black	M	44.8	14.1	32.9	15.5
	F	42.1	12.5	29.8	6.9
MexAm	M	49.9	16.0	39.0	27.7
	F	50.0	14.2	30.7	13.0
Hispanic			29.9		
Asian			29.2		
AmInd			31.2		

E. Secular trends, total cholesterol in mg/dL, age 12-17 (NCHS, NHLBI)

		1976-1980	1988-1994	1999-2002	2003-2004
White	M	63	163	155	156
	F	170	166	163	164
Black	M	171	165	166	161
	F	172	174	168	161

Adults

	1988-1994	1999-2002	2003-2004
Whites	206	204	202
Black	204	199	197
MexAm	205	202	201

9. Physical Activity

A. Prevalence 9th-12th graders meeting recommended levels of physical activity during past week, % of population (YRBS, 2005)

White	M	46.9
	F	30.2
Black	M	38.2
	F	21.3
Hispanic	M	39.0
	F	26.5

B. Prevalence of leisure time physical inactivity: Adults ≥18 years (BRFSS, 1999 and 2004)

		1994 %	2004 %
White	M	26.4	28.3
	F	28.3	21.6
Black	M	34.2	27.0
	F	45.7	33.9
Hispanic	M	37.5	32.5
	F	44.8	39.6
Asian	M	25.0	20.4
	F	31.5	24.0
AmInd	M	34.4	23.8
	F	36.3	31.8

10. Overweight and Obesity

A. Overweight in grades 9-12, by % (YRBS, 2005)

White	M	15.2
	F	8.2
Black	M	15.9
	F	16.1
Hispanic	M	21.3
	F	12.1

B. Prevalence of overweight and obesity, by %, age ≥20 years (2005 NHANES 2001-2004, NHIS 2005)

		Overweight + obesity	Obesity
White	M	71.0	30.2
	F	57.6	30.7
Black	M	67.0	30.8
	F	79.6	51.1
MexAm	M	74.6	29.1
	F	73.0	39.4
Hispanic	≥18 years	39.6	27.5
Asian	≥18 years	27.9	8.5
AmInd		38.6	37.6

Overweight=body mass index (BMI) ≥25 kg/m^2;
Obesity=BMI ≥30 kg/m^2

11. Diabetes Mellitus

A. Prevalence (2005, NHANES 1999-2004, NCHS, NHLBI)

Diabetes=fasting glucose ≥126 mg/dL;
Prediabetes=100-125 mg/dL

		Physician diagnosed and undiagnosed %	Prediabetes %
White	M	9.9	34.3
	F	7.3	21.6
Black	M	12.4	23.1
	F	15.5	20.5
MexAm	M	12.1	37.5
	F	14.0	22.6

References

1. *Circulation* 2008;117:325:e146.

2. Kleindorfer D, Broderick J, Khoury J, et al: The unchanging incidence and case-fatality of stroke in the 1990s: a population-based study. *Stroke* 2006;37:2473-2478.

12. Metabolic Syndrome

Prevalence % (NHANES, 1988-1994)

Criteria include three or more of the following:

- Fasting glucose ≥100 mg/dL
- Triglycerides ≥150 mg/dL
- Blood pressure ≥130 mm Hg systolic
  or ≥85 mm Hg diastolic
- Waist circumference ≥40 inches in men and
  ≥36 inches in women
- HDL-C <40 mg/dL in men and <50 mg/dL
  in women

White	M	24.3
	F	22.9
Black	M	13.9
	F	20.9
Hispanic	M	20.8
	F	27.2

3. Hertz RP, Unger AN, Cornell JA, et al: Racial disparities in hypertension prevalence, awareness, and management. *Arch Intern Med* 2005;165;2098-2104.

4. Hoffman JI, Kaplan S, Liberthson RR: Prevalence of congenital heart disease. *Am Heart J* 2004;147;425-439.

Guidelines Related to Special Populations

Class I Intervention useful and effective

IIa Evidence in favor of use

IIb Usefulness less well established

III Not effective or harmful

Level of Evidence

A Sufficient evidence from multiple clinical trials

B Limited evidence from single randomized trial or other studies

C Based on expert opinion, case studies, standard of care

A. Women[1]

Lifestyle/Major Risk Factor Interventions
( ) = Level of Evidence

High-risk=established coronary heart disease (CHD), cerebrovascular disease, peripheral arterial disease (PAD), abdominal aortic aneurysm, end-stage renal disease (ESRD), diabetes, or 10-year absolute risk >20%

Class I

- Cigarette smoking cessation (B)
- Cardiovascular or stroke rehabilitation after acute coronary syndrome (ACS), with angina, cerebrovascular event, PAD (A), or symptoms of heart failure (HF) with left-ventricular ejection fraction (LVEF) <40% (B)
- Dietary: saturated fat <10% calories, cholesterol <300 mg/dL, *trans* fats <1%, alcohol <2 drinks daily (B)
- Weight maintenance: body mass index (BMI) between 18.5–24.9 kg/m^2, waist circumference ≤35 inches (B)
- Blood pressure (BP): optimal <120/80 by lifestyle modifications, including weight control, limited salt intake, increased physical activity, alcohol moderation, and intake of fresh fruits, vegetables, and low-fat dairy products (B)
  Lifestyle + pharmacotherapy: with blood pressure ≥140/90 or ≥130/80 with diabetes or chronic kidney disease (CKD) (A)
- Lipids: use lifestyle approaches to aim for low-density lipoprotein cholesterol (LDL-C) <100 mg/dL, high-density lipoprotein cholesterol (HDL-C) >50 mg/dL, triglycerides (Tg) <150 mg/dL, and non-HDL-C <130 mg/dL (B)
  Use pharmacologic therapy with lifestyle modifications:
  1. in high-risk patient, to achieve an LDL-C level <100 mg/dL (A). Also in women with diabetes, other atherosclerotic cardiovascular disease (CVD), or 20% 10-year absolute risk >20% (B)
  2. if 10-year absolute risk is 10%-20%, if LDL-C is ≥130 mg/dL (B)
  3. even if 10-year absolute risk is <10%, if multiple risk factors are present and LDL-C ≥160 mg/dL (B)
  4. if LDL-C is ≥190 mg/dL no matter how few other risk factors are present (B)
- Diabetics: lifestyle and pharmacotherapy to keep glycosylated hemoglobin (HbA$_{1c}$) <7% (C)

Specific preventive drug interventions:

- Aspirin—high-risk women (75-325 mg/d) (A)
- Clopidogrel—high-risk women in which aspirin is contra-indicated (B)
- β-blockers—after myocardial infarction (MI), ACS, LV dysfunction ± heart failure, unless contraindicated (A)
- Angiotension-converting enzyme (ACE) inhibitors/angio-tension II receptor blockers (ARBs)—after MI with HF or LVEF ≤40%, or with diabetes (A). With these clinical findings, ARBs can be used if ACE inhibitors are contra-indicated (B)
- Aldosterone blockade—in women after MI with persistent LVEF ≤40% with symptomatic heart failure despite therapy with ACE inhibitors + β-blockers (B)

Class II

- Lipids: in high-risk women with low HDL-C or high non-HDL-C, after LDL-C goal is achieved, use niacin or fibrate therapy (IIa, B)

  Similarly, in women with multiple risk factors and 10-year absolute risk between 10%-20% (intermediate risk) (IIb, B)
- Omega-3 fatty acids: 850-1000 mg EPA or DHA with CHD and 2-4 g with high Tg (B)
- Depression: screen and treat when indicated (B)

Class III

- Menopausal therapy: hormonal therapy and selective estro-gen-receptor modulators neither for primary nor secondary prevention (A)
- Antioxidant supplements (vitamins E, C, and betacarotene): neither for primary nor secondary prevention (A)
- Folic acid: with or without B6 or B12 supplementation neither for primary nor secondary prevention (A)
- Aspirin: not for MI prevention in healthy women <65 years of age (B)

B. Children and Adolescents[2]

Disease stratification by risk

Step 1

- High risk: manifest CAD <30 years of age (clinical evidence)
  1. homozygous familial hypercholesterolemia (FH)
  2. diabetes mellitus, type 1
  3. chronic kidney disease/ESRD
  4. postorthostatic heart transplant
  5. Kawasaki disease with current coronary aneurysms

- Moderate risk: accelerated atherosclerosis (pathophysiologic evidence)
  1. heterozygous FH
  2. Kawasaki disease with regressed coronary aneurysms
  3. diabetes mellitus, type 2
  4. chronic inflammatory disease

- At risk: high-risk setting for accelerated atherosclerosis (epidemiologic evidence)
  1. post-cancer-treatment survivors
  2. congenital heart disease
  3. Kawasaki disease without coronary involvement

Step 2

Then evaluate standard cardiovascular risk factors.
  1. fasting lipid profile
  2. smoking history
  3. family history of early CAD in first-degree relative
  4. blood pressure
  5. BMI
  6. fasting glucose
  7. physical activity history

Step 3

If ≥2 comorbidities identified from step 2, increase risk category to next highest.

Step 4

Treatment goals

For all: Fasting glucose <100 mg/dL, HbA_{1c} <7%

- High risk:
  - BMI ≤85th percentile for age/sex
  - BP ≤90th percentile for age/sex
  - LDL-C ≤100 mg/dL
- Moderate risk:
  - BMI ≤90th percentile for age/sex
  - BP ≤95th percentile for age/sex
  - LDL-C ≤130 mg/dL
- At risk:
  - BMI ≤95th percentile for age/sex
  - BP ≤85th percentile for age/sex
  - LDL-C ≤160 mg/dL

Step 5

Initiate lifestyle modifications, but if goals are not met, consider medication, specific disease management for high-risk conditions

Specific treatment recommendations for disease management in high-risk category

- Homozygous FH
  1. LDL management: apheresis every 1-2 weeks plus statin and cholesterol absorption inhibitor
  2. Assess BMI, BP, and FG: lifestyle modifications for 6 months
  3. If goals are not achieved, initiate drug therapy

- Diabetes mellitus
    1. Intensive glucose management to maintain plasma glucose <100 mg/dL, HgA_{1c} <7%
    2. BMI, lipid intervention: lifestyle modifications
    3. Use statin if patient >10 years old for lipid intervention
    4. If BP >90th percentile for age/sex/height, restrict salt, increase physical activity
    5. If BP consistently >95th percentile for age/sex/height, start ACE inhibitor with goal <90th percentile or <130/80, whichever is lower
- CKD/ESRD
    1. Optimize renal failure management with dialysis/transplantation
    2. Manage BMI, BP, lipids, FG: lifestyle changes for 6 months, but if goals are not achieved, then initiate drug therapy (statins only if >10 years old)
- After heart transplantation
    1. Optimize antirejection therapy, treatment of CMV, routine evaluation by angiography/imaging
    2. Manage BMI, BP, lipids, FG: lifestyle changes + drug therapy, including statins, in all patients >1 year old
- Kawasaki disease with coronary aneurysms
    1. Antithrombotic therapy, physical activity restriction, ongoing perfusion evaluation by cardiologist
    2. Manage BMI, BP, lipids, FG, as above

General recommendations lifestyle modifications

- Growth/diet
    1. Diet education for all: <30% fat of total calories, saturated fat <10% of calories, cholesterol <300 mg/dL, avoid *trans* fats, adequate calories for growth
    2. Evaluate BMI: if BMI >85th percentile for age/sex/height, age-appropriate calorie training, with reduced calorie initiation and activity counseling

- Lipids (if elevated lipid levels)
    1. Diet: <30% fat calories, <7% calories from saturated fat, <200 mg/dL cholesterol, avoidance of *trans* fats for 6 months
- Smoking
    1. Parental smoking history at each visit; child smoking history beginning at age 10
    2. Active antismoking counseling for all; smoke-free home strongly recommended at each encounter
    3. Smoking cessation referral for smoking history
- Physical activity
    1. Goal: ≥1 hour active play per day; TV, computer, video game screen time ≤2 h/d
- High-risk lipid abnormalities[3]
    1. Fasting lipid profile with strong family history of premature CVD, and overweight or obesity in the child
    2. Overweight and obese children with lipid abnormalities should be screened for other aspects of metabolic syndrome (insulin resistance, type 2 diabetes, hypertension, central obesity)
    3. Risk factors that lower recommended cut point for LDL cholesterol for initiation of drug therapy:
        - Male gender
        - Strong family history of CVD or events
        - Overweight, obesity, metabolic syndrome
        - Associated low HDL-C, high Tg, small, dense LDL
        - Other conditions with an increased risk: diabetes, HIV infection, systemic lupus erythematosus, organ transplantation, survival of childhood cancer, hypertension, smoking and passive smoke exposure
        - Novel and emerging risk factors: Lp(a), homocysteine, s-CRP

4. Drug therapy for children ≥10 years (after menarche in females) after a 6- to 12- month trial of fat- and cholesterol-restricted diet
5. Drug therapy if:
   - LDL-C remains ≥190 mg/dL
   - LDL-C remains ≥160 mg/dL and:
   (a) history of premature CVD
   (b) ≥other risk factors present after vigorous attempts to control these other risk factors
6. Treatment goal:
   - Minimal LDL-C <130 mg/dL
   - Ideal LDL-C <110 mg/dL
- High blood pressure[4]

Categories:

1. Normal: <90th percentile for age, sex, height
2. Prehypertension: 90th to <95th percentile or >120/80 if <90th–<95th percentile
3. Stage 1 hypertension: 95th-99th percentile + 5 mm Hg
4. Stage 2 hypertension: >99th percentile + 5 mm Hg

Interventions:

Therapeutic lifestyle changes (categories 2, 3, 4)

1. Weight management counseling if overweight
2. Physical activity
3. Dietary management

Drug Therapy:

1. Symptomatic hypertension
2. Secondary hypertension
3. Hypertensive target organ damage
4. Diabetes (types 1 and 2)
5. Persistent hypertension despite lifestyle changes
6. Stage 2 hypertension

Acceptable pharmacologic agents:
1. ACE inhibitors
2. ARBs
3. β-blockers
4. Calcium channel blockers
5. Diuretics

Goal: Reduction to <95th percentile for age/sex/height; if concurrent conditions, <90th percentile

Secondary causes of hypertension:

Endocrine:
1. Adrenal hyperplasia
2. Cushing syndrome
3. Hyperaldosteronism
4. Hyperthyroidism

Renal:
1. Chronic renal failure
2. Liddle syndrome
3. Polycystic kidney disease

Oncologic:
1. Neuroblastoma
2. Neurofibromatosis
3. Pheochromocytoma
4. Wilms tumor

Vascular:
1. Coarctation of aorta
2. Collagen vascular disease
3. Renal artery stenosis
4. Williams syndrome

Other:
1. Sleep apnea (adenotonsillar hypertrophy)
2. Tuberous sclerosis
3. Turner syndrome

Target organ damage:
1. LVH (echo) (>51 g/m^2)
2. Renal insufficiency, albuminuria
3. Retinal abnormalities

C. African-Americans[5]

With multiple cardiovascular risk factors; risk factors to consider:

- Systolic BP ≥130 mm Hg, diastolic blood pressure ≥85 mm Hg
- Left ventricular hypertrophy (LVH)
- Family history of type 2 diabetes
- History of gestational diabetes
- Birth of infant >9 lb
- Fasting blood glucose 110-125 mg/dL
- Serum triglyceride level ≥150 mg/dL
- Serum LDL-C ≥140 mg/dL
- Serum HDL-C <40 mg/dL
- Central obesity
- Waist/hip ratio >0.8 (women), >0.95 (men)
- BMI >27 kg/m^2
- Cigarette smoking
- Serum homocysteine >15 μmol/L
- Serum plasma activator inhibitor-1 (PAI-1) >15 IU/L

- History of clot formation
- Polycystic ovary syndrome
- Acanthosis nigricans
- Gout or serum uric acid >8.5 mg/dL

The guidelines recommend aggressive management if multiple risk factors are present based on recommendations of the National Cholesterol Education Program (for lipids) and the Joint National Committee 7 Report on the Treatment of Hypertension. Diabetes should be treated based on American Diabetes Association guidelines. Smoking cessation, dietary intervention for weight reduction, lipid modifications, salt intake reduction, and physical activity are important adjuncts to risk factor interventions.

References

1. Mosca L, Banks CL, Benjamin EJ, et al for the Expert Panel/Writing Group: Evidence-based guidelines for cardiovascular disease prevention in women (2007 update). *Circulation* 2007;115: 1481-1501.

2. Kavey RW: Cardiovascular risk reduction in high-risk pediatric patients. *Circulation* 2006;114:2710-2738.

3. McCrindle BW, Urbina EM, Dennison BA, et al: Drug therapy of high-risk lipid abnormalities in children and adolescents: a scientific statement from the American Heart Association Atherosclerosis, Hypertension, and Obesity in Youth Committee, Council of Cardiovascular Disease in the Young, with the Council on Cardiovascular Nursing. *Circulation* 2007;115:1948-1967.

4. Fourth Report on the Diagnosis, Evaluation, and Treatment of High Blood Pressure in Children and Adolescents. *Pediatrics* 2004;112:555-576.

5. Williams RA, Flack JM, Gavin JR 3rd, et al: Guidelines for management of high-risk African Americans with multiple cardiovascular risk factors: recommendations of an expert consensus panel. *Ethn Dis* 2007;17:214-220.

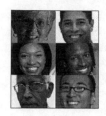

Index

NOTES

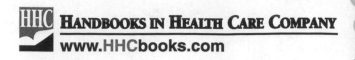
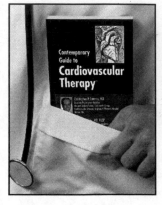